Miracle Cures

ALSO BY JEAN CARPER

Stop Aging Now!
Food—Your Miracle Medicine
The Food Pharmacy
The Food Pharmacy Guide to Good Eating

Miracle Cures

DRAMATIC *new* SCIENTIFIC DISCOVERIES
REVEALING THE *healing* POWERS OF *herbs,*
vitamins, AND OTHER *natural* REMEDIES

Jean Carper

HarperCollins*Publishers*

HarperCollins books may be purchased for educational, business, or sales promotional use. For information please write: Special Markets Department, HarperCollins Publishers, Inc., 10 East 53rd Street, New York, NY 10022.

FIRST EDITION

Designed by Laura Lindgren

Library of Congress Cataloging-in-Publication Data

Carper, Jean.
   Miracle cures : dramatic new scientific discoveries revealing the
   healing powers of herbs, vitamins, and other natural remedies /
   by Jean Carper. — 1st ed.
       p.   cm.
   Includes index.
   ISBN 0-06-018372-1
   1. Naturopathy.   2. Herbs—Therapeutic use.   3. Dietary
   supplements.   I. Title
   RZ440.C336   1997
   615.5'35—dc21   97-13747

97 98 99 00 01 ❖/RRD 10 9 8 7 6 5 4 3 2 1

To all the Carpers

CONTENTS

CONTENTS

ACKNOWLEDGMENTS

As always, I would like to thank the many scientists, researchers, doctors, and other health professionals who shared with me their research and expertise, making this book possible. In particular, Mark Blumenthal, executive director, American Botanical Council; Dr. Donald Brown, director of Natural Products Research Consultants; Luke Bucci, Ph.D., expert on natural products; Jerry Cott, Ph.D., National Institute of Mental Health; James Duke, Ph.D., formerly with the U.S. Department of Agriculture and the author of many books on medicinal plants; Norman Farnsworth, Ph.D., University of Illinois at Chicago; Balz Frei, Ph.D., Boston University; Turan Itil, M.D., clinical professor of psychiatry, New York University; Tricia LeFebvre, Primary Services International; Rob McCaleb, the Herb Research Institute; Dr. Michael Murray, author and national authority on natural remedies; Richard Passwater, Ph.D., author of many books on natural remedies; Norman Rosenthal, M.D., National Institute of Mental Health; Norman Salem, Ph.D., National Institute of Mental Health; Stephen Sinatra, M.D., assistant clinical professor, University of Connecticut; Daniel Tucker, M.D., Good Samaritan Medical Center, West Palm Beach, Florida; Varro Tyler, Ph.D., professor emeritus of pharmacognosy, Purdue University; Marcia Zimmerman, a California consultant, who was a primary source on OPCs.

ACKNOWLEDGMENTS

I would especially like to double-thank Mark Blumenthal for his expert comments in reviewing sections of the book dealing with botanical medicines before publication. Also, I owe a special debt to Varro Tyler, Ph.D., a distinguished authority on botanical medicines, who patiently and expertly answered all my questions and sat for numerous interviews that contributed greatly to this book.

Dozens of people added to the vitality and importance of this book by sharing personal experiences of their "miracle cures." They are mentioned throughout the book, sometimes by actual name, and sometimes by a pseudonym at their request, to protect their privacy.

This book could not have been written without the enormous contribution of two researchers who tracked down patients, doctors, and research studies: Brenda Turner and Peggy Noonan. Special thanks to Brenda for devoting her full four-month sabbatical from her job as an editor at *USA Weekend* to making this book happen.

As always, thanks to both my publisher, Gladys Justin Carr, and my agent, Raphael Sagalyn, for seeing the potential of this book and making its realization possible.

It is hard to imagine writing a book without the expert editorial input of my longtime friend, television producer Thea Flaum, who knows how much I treasure and respect her advice.

This book will educate the reader about natural drugs, remedies, treatments, medicines, cures, and "dietary supplements." It is based on the personal experiences, research, and observations of the author, who is not a medical or naturopathic doctor. This book is intended to be informational and by no means should be considered a substitute for advice from a medical or health professional, who should be consulted by the reader in matters relating to his or her health and particularly in respect to any symptoms that may require medical attention. While every effort has been made to ensure that drug selections and dosages are in accordance with current recommendations and practices, because of ongoing research and other factors, the reader is cautioned to check with a health professional about specific recommendations. Anyone with a known disease or serious health condition or who is taking prescription medications should especially seek professional medical advice before taking the natural remedies described in this book. There could be interactions between the natural remedies and other drugs. Also it should be noted that all dosages discussed in this book apply to adults, not children, unless otherwise stated. The author and publisher expressly disclaim responsibility for any adverse effects arising from the use or application of the information contained in this book.

Searching for the Truth About Natural Remedies

I went not only to the doctors, but also to barbers, bath-keepers, learned physicians, women, and magicians who pursue the art of healing; I went to alchemists, monasteries, to nobles and the common folk, to the experts and the simple.

PARACELSUS (1443–1541)

This book is a personal investigation into the validity of natural drugs, remedies, treatments, medicines, and cures, and their accelerating integration into mainstream medicine. While writing and researching the book, I was constantly surprised and impressed by the vigor of this national trend. The incorporation of natural medicinals into conventional medicine is happening much faster than most people realize. And it will eventually have a dramatic beneficial impact, if it has not already, on all of us personally and on the quality and cost of our health care. We are talking about major changes and reforms in a basic structure of all medical systems, from ancient to modern: the appropriate use of drugs to overcome sickness.

Here's what surprised me most:

- The intensity and persistence of people in seeking safer, effective cures outside conventional treatments, even in the face of resistance from establishment medicine.

- The willingness, even eagerness, of leading doctors and scientists at the very core of modern scientific medicine—at the National Institutes of Health and prestigious research and academic centers—to explore the potential of unconventional remedies.
- The mounting scientific evidence supporting the validity and safety of natural remedies.
- The extensive study and use of such natural remedies among mainstream doctors in other countries, especially Germany.
- The utter chaos of government regulations regarding the use of natural medicines, which is reflected in a consumer nightmare in the marketplace.

When I started this book, I knew, of course, that Americans are embarked on a new direction in seeking solutions for their own health problems. But I had no idea of the strength and pervasiveness of this quest at all strata of society. It was inspiring to talk to people from all walks of life who had developed their own personal health agendas, expending enormous energy to find alternative treatments when they felt mainstream medicine had failed them by providing ineffective treatments or treatments that carried more risk than they wanted to take. Dozens of people openly expressed sentiments ranging from discouragement and resentment to enthusiasm and hope about their personal predicaments. I collected case histories and personal stories from truck drivers, boat captains, airline pilots, doctors, lawyers, secretaries, librarians, journalists, factory workers, computer operators, biochemists, psychologists, teachers, athletes, pharmacologists, botanists, and legislators. Each one had a story of how he or she had suffered and been helped by what is called "alternative" or "complementary" medicine—something not typically offered by conventional medicine.

Their exuberance over their successes affirmed the title of this book. Virtually all of them used the term "miracle cure" in recounting their experiences. Even doctors, I found, often used the word "miracle" in describing what happened when a patient suddenly got well after taking a natural remedy. The word "miracle" is defined in dictionaries as "a wonder, a marvel," as well as an act or happening that departs from the laws of nature. Thus, when a person recovers after taking a natural substance, the event is so incongruous with conventional medical expectations that the first words of surprise and overwhelming gratitude are typically: "It's a miracle cure." We often say the same thing about conventional treatments that amaze us.

You may also be surprised to learn what the word "cure" means medically. It is not a complete and permanent medical resolution, as most people think. "Cure" actually means, according to *Dorland's Medical Dictionary*: "The course of treatment of any disease, the successful treatment of a disease or wound, a system of treating diseases, a medicine effective in treating a disease."

My own consciousness has been dramatically raised while writing this book. My own miracle cures have not been for life-threatening diseases, but have nevertheless been of major importance to me. About two years ago I began taking glucosamine sulfate, at the suggestion of Dr. Michael Murray, a nationally known naturopathic doctor, to treat the beginnings of osteoarthritis in my hands. I am convinced it has helped save me from much distress by slowing progression of the disease and relieving pain. The sharp stabs of pain in the joints of my fingers and thumbs have virtually disappeared (they came back only when I temporarily stopped taking glucosamine), and my grip for opening jars and holding a tennis racket is much firmer and stronger than it was. I have recommended all the remedies in this book to friends and family. My brother and one of my sisters, both of whom suffered heart attacks, take 200 milligrams of coQ–10 daily. Another sister's cholesterol plunged after she took the grapefruit fiber detailed in this book. I have handed out more than one kava pill to friends when they are anxious. My niece is taking feverfew to prevent migraine headaches. My brother-in-law is taking St. John's wort instead of Prozac. My ninety-two-year-old mother has been taking ginkgo biloba for two years, since her memory began to falter. I think it has helped her greatly.

Doing the research for this book was formidable and quite different from the research for the other nineteen books I have written, most on related health and nutrition subjects. In researching other books, I found that much of the medical literature was readily available. It was mostly a matter of gathering it, analyzing it, checking it out with many well-credentialed scientific authorities, and translating it into concepts and advice that can be understood by readers. Gathering information on natural remedies, however, was like sailing on uncharted waters. Although the amount of research appearing in mainstream medical journals has recently picked up dramatically, much of the research on natural remedies is in foreign journals, some not translated into English or not reported in mainstream medical databases. Nor are there the familiar touchstones of medical expertise in academic centers to confirm and illuminate the facts that are emerging. Instead, the people who know most about the clinical use of natural remedies are practitioners and patients, spread throughout the country. And much of the research in the United States is being conducted in scattered fashion by individual interested doctors and scientists, rarely under the usual centralized auspices of the National Institutes of Health. Without a bedrock of established and familiar sources, research was a matter of tracking down leads from many divergent sources, based on tips from scientists, doctors, and patients.

My file drawers are full of information not appearing in this book. In the beginning, with the help of two wonderful researchers, I jumped in to take a closer look at practically every natural remedy we had read or heard about. At places like the big Expo Health Fair trade shows in Baltimore, we collected shopping bags full of information on hundreds of products claiming to be natural remedies. We read dozens of magazines, tracked down every legitimate-sounding lead on people who reputedly had used natural medicines successfully. We scoured the Internet for cases and information. We did database searches on the purported remedies in both the popular press and the scientific journals. We talked to pioneering scientists who were reportedly using and researching a variety of natural substances. We talked to leading herbal authorities, naturopathic doctors, professors at universities, and highly regarded industry representatives who make the natural remedies in the United States and in Europe.

It was exhilarating, inspiring, informative, enlightening, and often discouraging and disheartening. As a mainstream medical journalist, I was both wildly enthusiastic about and sometimes appalled by the claims for some remedies. Often I was saddened and irritated by a closed-minded medical establishment's unwillingness even to hear about or try a perfectly safe, medically tested botanical medicine, such as feverfew to prevent migraines. Other times, I understood some of the skepticism and cynicism surrounding natural remedies, especially when the claims were so wild, the products so irrational, and the prices so outrageously exploitative.

In the end, after I had sought out patients, doctors, and scientists for their opinions, I had to make judgments, based on my best overall appraisal of a few hundred or more natural remedies. Which to include in this book? Which seemed best? Which had the most scientific support? Which were leading authorities in the field using and recommending? Which were safe? Which were attracting the most mainstream scientific attention as most promising for future use? Which would I myself use personally or recommend to friends and family—because of or even regardless of substantial mainstream evidence of effectiveness?

The last consideration was the deciding factor for me—whether I, knowing what I know, would enthusiastically and comfortably use a natural remedy myself and recommend it to those I care about. That is the main rationale to explain why certain remedies are detailed in this book and others are not.

As I whittled away at the long list of candidates to write about, I discarded some remedies because I could find no authentic value in them; others seemed too risky or just plain irresponsible or silly. I admit that a few remedies got into the book because of my respect for the personalities who use them—Dr. Jim Duke, the colorful botanist; Dr. James Gordon, a pioneering doctor; and Tom Harkin, a U.S. senator with the power and interest to help determine the future of natural medicines in this country. All of them are responsible, intelligent, and even wise in their commonsense approach to trusting their own experiences of natural remedies. Sometimes the validity of a remedy is in the successful use, not in a controlled scientific study, as Dr. Gordon points out.

In short, this is a book about what many scientists, doctors, and patients are saying and doing about natural medicines and what you can learn from them. Unquestionably, in my mind, there is new, exciting, and mounting evidence that should rally Americans to embrace many of these natural remedies sensibly. Not to give them serious consideration is to remain unenlightened. Here's why, according to what I discovered while writing this book:

- Herbs, vitamins, and other natural remedies do work, according to many patients, doctors, and scientific researchers.
- They are safe if chosen and used appropriately.
- They are often as effective and safe as, or more effective and safer than, conventional mainstream medical drugs or treatments.
- They are usually far less expensive.
- They have accomplished "miracle cures" for many people, and they may do the same for you or someone you care about.

This book, I hope, will inspire you to try them.

The Revolution Is Here:

What You
Need to Know to Join

Do those potions you see in health food stores, drugstores, supermarkets, mail order outlets, and discount chains really work? Is there any scientific validity to their seemingly extravagant promises? And, most of all, will these natural drugs help cure you or someone you care about of minor vexatious illness, such as flu and low energy, or major debilitating and life-threatening diseases, such as heart failure, cancer, arthritis, diabetes, cirrhosis, depression, and mental deterioration?

You might ask those same questions of millions of people around the world who have successfully used natural remedies. The resounding answer is yes. Some Americans might say the same thing. However, sadly, America generally is far behind other countries in the use of natural medicines, because of a lack of knowledge about their scientific validity and a failure of our medical profession and the government to properly evaluate and endorse their use. Consequently, you and millions of other Americans are being deprived of the opportunity to choose natural treatments in place of strong, often harmful and expensive pharmaceutical drugs. Yet, such natural medicines could reduce or eliminate some of the harsh consequences of our conventional treatments, in terms of both human and economic suffering. At least, we should explore the incredible potential healing powers of those natural remedies that have been widely tested and extensively used with governmental approval in many foreign countries, including Germany, France, and England—all countries with impeccable scientific and medical standards. Unless we do, we cannot say that we have access to the best medical care in the world.

Fortunately, the attitude toward natural treatments is rapidly changing in the United States. More scientific information on natural medicines is coming into the country; prestigious scientists and doctors here are increasingly testing and using such natural remedies and comparing their effectiveness and safety with pharmaceutical drugs. And Americans are embracing the natural medications and so-called "alternative" or "complementary" treatments with enthusiasm.

It's no secret that the American public is turning in droves to nontraditional remedies. A startling 1993 report in the trusted *New England Journal of Medicine* showed that one-third of Americans use nonconventional treatments, spending $10.8 billion yearly, but most never tell their doctors. A 1997 *Prevention* magazine survey of the general public (not just its readers) found that about one-third of adult Americans, or 60 million, say they frequently use "herbal remedies." Even people in the industry were surprised. "Herbs are becoming more mainstream much faster than we ever expected," said Mary Burnett, spokesperson for the Council for Responsible Nutrition, a Washington, D.C., trade association for the nutritional supplement industry.

Yes, herbal remedies, botanical medicines, and natural

drugs of all kinds, available anywhere without restriction or prescription, are being embraced by Americans. "Medical experts say that over the past ten years, more people have been turning to more kinds of alternative therapies than ever before," wrote *New York Times* science reporter Gina Kolata in June 1996. Some see this movement as "a return to our roots," a desire for natural medicines used by our ancestors. But it is also driven by a seemingly unstoppable coalition of social and economic forces—soaring health care costs, a growing disillusionment with the limitations and hazards of high-tech medicine, increasing concerns about adverse effects from pharmaceutical drugs, and a reaction against an authoritarian medical system in which doctors appear to play God. In such circumstances, natural remedies seem ideal solutions; they are usually far cheaper, are perceived as much safer, and give patients increased freedom to direct their own health care.

Some mainstream doctors fear the growing use of alternative therapies, but others believe it makes social and scientific sense. They are open to the idea that other cultures and countries may have valid ways of curing diseases that could be good for Americans. We love to say we have the best health care in the world, but that is debatable, and even so, it is costing us a fortune—a situation that threatens to worsen as our population ages. Some health authorities believe we are squandering our national resources needlessly, even as we fail to control our epidemic of chronic diseases, including heart disease and cancer. It's just possible we can learn something about the human complexities and traditions involved in healing, not only from Asian healers but also from scientifically minded Western physicians in Germany and France, where natural remedies are treated as legitimate mainstream medicines, not as aberrations of an unenlightened populace.

One reason people turn to "alternative" medicine is that our mainstream medical system is failing. The fact is, we are in the midst of an epidemic of inadequately treated chronic illness. Sixty million Americans have hypertension, 40 million suffer from arthritis, and 23 million of us have migraine headaches. A million Americans each year are being diagnosed with cancer, and close to 40 percent of us will, at one point or another, have this terrifying and often deadly disease. The prevalence of asthma, multiple sclerosis, chronic fatigue, immune deficiency syndrome, HIV, and a host of other debilitating conditions is increasing. Conventional biomedicine—so strikingly successful in the treatment of overwhelming infections, surgical and medical emergencies, and congenital defects, has been unable to stem the tide of these conditions.—James Gordon, M.D., a Washington, D.C., psychiatrist and a clinical professor at the Georgetown University School of Medicine

MAINSTREAM MEDICAL BREAKTHROUGHS

Indeed, the idea that natural substances have a genuine place in modern medicine is spreading, attracting advocates in high places in the United States—at academic and governmental medical centers, such as Harvard and the National Institutes of Health. The credibility of natural therapies is infiltrating mainstream medicine. Many studies of impeccable quality showing the value of natural medicines are now appearing in prestigious scientific journals such as *The Lancet*, the *British Medical Journal*, the *New England Journal of Medicine*, the *Journal of the American Medical Association*, and the journals of the American Heart Association, as well as in leading German and Japanese publications. Using rigorous scientific standards, many prestigious investigators at leading research centers are testing natural substances to treat some of our most serious diseases and even comparing the effectiveness and safety of these natural drugs with conventional pharmaceutical drugs. Often they find strong pharmacological activity in nature's remedies. Sometimes the natural agents are fully as effective as the hard-hitting "drugs of choice" of mainstream medicine. Usually the natural medicines are much safer, often having little or no toxicity and few if any significant adverse side effects.

This prompts one to ask whether our concept of which treatment should be called "alternative" is topsy-turvy. In standard American medical practice, conventional hard-hitting drugs are always the first choice, with unconventional remedies considered a last-resort "alternative." Isn't it more logical to try a more benign remedy first most of the time, and then proceed to a stronger, more risky remedy as the "alternative" if the first does not work? Many more doctors and patients than ever before think that makes sense, and their thinking is reflected in changes that are bringing natural remedies to mainstream attention.

Witness the establishment of the Office of Alternative Medicine at the National Institutes of Health in 1993. The office, though underfunded, is committed to research on "alternative" therapies and has given grants to leading institutions and practitioners to study the efficacy and safety of botanical medicines, among other nonconventional treatments. In June 1996 a blue-ribbon panel of the Office of Alternative Medicine urged medical and nursing schools to start teaching alternative medicine. Dr. Wayne Jonas, director of the office, said about forty medical schools around the country have added courses on alternative medicine, including top-rated Harvard and Johns Hopkins.

A PHARMACEUTICAL TRAGEDY

Part of the search for more natural benign medicines is triggered by growing concern over the hazards of our current pharmaceutical climate that dispenses so many drugs with dreadful side effects. Drug reactions are a national tragedy. Sidney M. Wolfe, M.D., head of Public Citizen's Health Research Group, laid out the situation in a February 1996 newsletter called *Worst Pills, Best Pills News*.

> Unquestionably, the U.S. drug industry manufactures countless products which can greatly benefit patients. But, in their zeal to make as much money as possible—in 1995, the pharmaceutical industry led all other industries in profitability—many drugs are over-promoted in a way which overstates their benefits and understates their risks. The $10 billion per year of often dangerously misleading drug promotional expenditures fit hand in glove with inadequate education of doctors about drugs and, together, place you and your family at risk of serious adverse drug reactions. Each year, for example, more than 1 million Americans have to be hospitalized because of adverse drug reactions—61,000 people get drug-induced parkinsonism, 16,000 people have injurious auto accidents caused by prescription drugs, 163,000 people have drug-induced or drug-worsened memory loss and there are 32,000 people with hip fractures caused by drug-induced falls.
>
> Most—at least two-thirds—of these adverse reac-

tions are preventable. All too often a "worst pill" was prescribed when a safer, equally effective one would have done just as well, or two relatively safe—if given alone—drugs were prescribed together causing a life threatening interaction between them.

The excessive, often indiscriminate dispensing of such prescription drugs has also made us a nation of unwitting junkies. Although we spend millions to stamp out illegal drugs that destroy human beings, our major addiction problem stems not from heroin or cocaine or other illegal drugs, but from legal prescription drugs, many given out by doctors without concern for addiction. A new study released in 1997 found that in 1995 more than 6 million Americans abused prescription drugs, such as the widely used antianxiety drug Xanax. This is far more than abused heroin and cocaine together. The consequences of such legal accidental addiction can be awful, destroying the lives of people who were crying for help to treat a legitimate problem such as panic attacks, and ended up either hopelessly addicted or in detox programs.

The truth is, there are far less dangerous drugs being successfully used every day throughout the world to treat diseases. It is almost a criminal act of negligence not to pursue the use of such natural substances in the United States. Yet there are many obstacles.

THE SORRY STATE IN THE UNITED STATES

When you buy natural drugs at health food stores, drugstores, and supermarkets, you are on your own in a circus atmosphere of bizarre government regulation. Our natural remedies cannot be advertised or sold as such, but are marketed as food—as "dietary supplements." Thus you cannot even tell exactly what the product is designed to treat. The labels are forbidden to make "health claims," but may make only vague and meaningless claims that a product affects a "structure or function" of the body, such as "good for the eyes" or "good for the circulation."

Happily, some manufacturers are responsible, turn out terrific products, and conscientiously try to inform the public, although they are hamstrung by federal prohibitions on making health and therapeutic claims. However, some of the criticism of the makers and sellers of natural substances is unfortunately valid. Some products are poorly conceived and poorly made. Some are mishmash combinations of herbs that make no sense but are contrived to create a "unique" or overpriced product. Some contain so little active stuff that they are worthless. Some are outrageously overpriced and deceptively labeled and promoted. And you can't rely on sales personnel to enlighten you. Although some clerks are well informed, many are not, and contribute to the public ignorance.

Mainly to blame for this dismal state of affairs is a disastrous regulatory system that discourages the development, testing, and manufacture of high-quality natural remedies. Most of the high-quality natural remedies in health food stores, such as coenzyme Q-10, St. John's wort, echinacea, milk thistle, and ginkgo—are made in foreign countries, mainly Germany and Japan, and repackaged for American consumption. Ironically, some of the raw materials are native to this country—saw palmetto is a prime example—and are exported for processing into natural drugs, because our system discourages businesses here from doing it.

It's difficult to understand how our regulations concerning natural medicines got into such a mess. Suffice it to say that it happened over a period of years and of late there has been some strange maneuvering involving a mutually antagonistic FDA and Congress, which resulted in some halfway regulatory measures but not full reforms.

WHY NOT DO RESEARCH?

Another problem is inherent in our legal wrangling over natural substances to be used as medicines—the patent situation. Some people ask: If natural remedies are so good, why aren't more studies done in this country to prove it? Why don't drug or supplement companies do such studies? The answer is simple. There is little or no economic incentive for American companies to spend money to test a botanical medicine because the financial rewards are small to nonexistent. Nature owns the patent on most of these medicinals, which means that nobody can get an exclusive patent to manufacture and market them. It's not worthwhile for a company to do expensive tests of a natural remedy that is available to all competitors. Pharmaceutical drugs are so profitable because their exclusivity is guaranteed by a patent. Nobody can steal the results of the company's financial investment in researching such drugs. With natural medicines, anybody can steal anything.

Further, companies do not want to confront the FDA bureaucracy to try to get approval of a natural remedy as a new drug: It costs millions of dollars and takes years; the natural drug may not be approved; and if it is approved, it still can't be sold for the high prices commanded by synthetic pharmaceuticals. Sometimes companies can get natural medicines approved by the FDA as over-the-counter drugs. But in general our system thoroughly discourages the generation of and dissemination of knowledge about natural medicines.

In short, the American marketplace for natural cures is a nightmare. Health food stores and drugstores are awash in products of unknown quality, effectiveness, and safety. But the good news is, it doesn't have to be that way. It is not that way in many other countries. A shining example is Germany. That's why many of the high-quality, well-tested natural remedies sold in this country come from Germany. Many leading authorities, such as Dr. Varro Tyler, professor emeritus of pharmacognosy (the medicinal study of plants) at Purdue University, say we should upgrade our regulatory system to deal with nature's medicines the way the Germans do.

Dr. Tyler, in his excellent book *Herbs of Choice*, blames our dismal failure to regulate herbal remedies properly for a widespread consumer catastrophe. "We have the worst regulations in the world with respect to these products. Consequently, the customer cannot be assured of anything. The lack of sound information and the abundance of misinformation in the herbal field cause normally well-informed critical consumers to become lost in a jungle of exaggerated claims and unsubstantiated assertions."

THEY DO IT RIGHT IN GERMANY

Much of the twentieth-century scientific knowledge about the amazing powers of plant medicines comes from Germany, where the scientific and governmental attitude toward such remedies is entirely positive. In that country botanical medicines are approved as over-the-counter drugs by a government body known as Commission E, which is similar to our Food and Drug Administration. Doctors are also given strict guidelines on which natural remedies to prescribe for which conditions, and their expected effectiveness and safety. The natural substances are meticulously manufactured to pharmaceutical standards and clearly labeled as to their approved uses and doses, possible side effects, toxicity, and contraindications.

Established in 1978, Commission E examines all the modern scientific evidence available on herbal remedies, including well-conducted studies on humans, and also takes into consideration the historic traditional use of the botanical medicine. Commission E has issued about 300 monographs on herbal medicines, 200 of which it has approved as reasonably effective and absolutely safe. The standard of proof of efficacy is not as strict as the double-blind human studies required by our FDA for pharmaceutical drugs. However, the German Commission E insists on proof that the drug is effective for certain conditions, as shown by research and traditional usage, and, moreover, that it cannot be harmful when used as designated.

This regulatory mechanism allows the public to have confidence in and knowledge about botanical medicines for sale in Germany. They can readily buy the remedies over the counter in retail stores. But physicians, all of whom must study botanical medicines in medical school, also regularly write prescriptions for them. The reason: If a German doctor specifically recommends or prescribes the medicine, it can be paid for by the government. Thus patients have an economic incentive for getting a prescription for over-the-counter herbal remedies. In fact, according to a new survey, 80 percent of German physicians prescribe phyto (plant) medicines; such natural drugs account for 27 percent of all over-the-counter medicines sold in Germany. Most popular are ginkgo, garlic, echinacea, and Asian ginseng.

Because of Germany's superior regulatory system, it consistently turns out the very best quality herbal medicines. If you want good, safe natural remedies, backed up by research, you need regulatory mechanisms that support superb testing, evaluation of safety and efficacy, quality control of products, accurate labeling, and information on proper doses, use, and adverse effects, says Dr. Varro Tyler.

The quality of research on herbal remedies is so outstanding in Germany, says Dr. Tyler, precisely because its government's regulatory system actively encourages natural remedies, making research worthwhile for consumers and doctors and profitable for companies that make and test herbal products. Much of the high-quality testing of natural remedies used in the United States and throughout the world, including St. John's wort (an antidepressant herb), valerian (an antianxiety herb), and echinacea (an antiviral herb), has been conducted in Germany.

In Germany the scientific-regulatory establishment simply has a different attitude toward the possibilities of natural remedies. While we focus almost entirely on strong pharmaceuticals, German scientists also constantly investigate natural alternatives. For example, in 1994 our FDA approved the first pharmaceutical drug—tacrine—for treating dementia and Alzheimer's disease. The drug is somewhat effective but has toxic side effects that limit its use. That same year, Germany's Commission E approved ginkgo biloba, a standardized extract from the leaves of the ginkgo tree, as a treatment for dementia and Alzheimer's. It works—some leading American investigators find it more promising than tacrine—and has virtually no toxicity or side effects. Ginkgo is also approved in Germany for "cerebral insufficiency," another name for age-related mental decline. Unfortunately, much of the scientific information generated in Germany remains unavailable to American doctors and consumers; some of it is in German medical journals and has not been translated into

English or included in the large database at the National Library of Medicine, which is the standard resource for American medicine. Recently, however, because of a surging interest in botanical medicines, more German studies are becoming available in the United States, and the American Botanical Council has published an English translation of all the Commission E monographs on herbal medicines. Dr. Tyler and others hail these monographs as the most complete and reliable scientific compendium of evidence on botanical medicines in the Western world. (See page 282 for how to obtain it.)

So many of our good American plant drugs (such as echinacea and saw palmetto) had to be researched in Europe because we don't have reasonable laws and regulations here that promote the scientific development of botanicals. I personally think that's just an utter tragedy.—Dr. Varro Tyler, dean emeritus of the School of Pharmacy at Purdue University and leading authority on plant medicines

WHO'S ON CALL?

In many other countries, if you have a question about a natural remedy, you can get a valid answer from your doctor or pharmacist. Plenty of trained professionals oversee the rational dispersal of natural drugs. In Germany physicians and pharmacists are required to pass tests on their knowledge of botanical medicines. They regularly prescribe and dispense natural drugs and can answer questions about their benefits and safety. Truly, one of the big dilemmas in the United States is that we have no reliable medical enclave that individuals can rely on and trust to give advice on natural remedies.

Unless you are lucky, you do not have a doctor, a pharmacist, or another health professional who knows much about such substances. "If they didn't learn it in medical school—and they don't—they think it's not true," says Dr. Daniel Tucker, a board-certified allergist and internist at Good Samaritan Medical Center in Palm Beach, Florida. Dr. Tucker is an excellent example of a well-credentialed physician who is adapting to the changing climate and coming integration of conventional and alternative medicine to form "complementary" medicine. He uses all the appropriate conventional medicines, but when a safer, better, less expensive remedy may work, such as feverfew for migraines, he suggests that, too. Many enlightened medical doctors are integrating "alternative" medicine into their practices. But, unfortunately, the only way most people find such doctors is by word of mouth.

The nation's best current repository of reliable information on natural remedies consists of naturopathic doctors, who carry an "N.D." behind their names. They are a formidable force in the Northwest, where the nation's two accredited naturopathic medical schools are located—Bastyr University in Seattle and the National College of Naturopathic Medicine in Portland, Oregon. Such naturopathic doctors, after an undergrad pre-med education, attend the naturopathic medical schools, where they take about ten times more classroom hours in therapeutic nutrition than do doctors in traditional medical schools. As of early 1997 twelve states licensed naturopathic doctors. In Washington state a new law forces insurance companies to pay for naturopathic treatments. The first complementary medical clinic opened in Seattle in 1997, merging natural and conventional treatments. Clinic patients can choose one or the other, or both types of treatment. It is managed by Bastyr University.

RED FLAGS, RED HERRINGS, AND LEGITIMATE CONCERNS

Much misinformation has been disseminated and many false alarms have been sounded in this country about the use of natural remedies. Some concerns are legitimate and deserve attention; some are simply innocent misunderstandings; some stem from a reluctance to tolerate change in the status quo or the medical establishment; some come from sheer ignorance and a few from unreasonable hostility, sometimes related to threats to an individual's position or status. For example, some scientists fear that their government grant money will be "misdirected" to study "quack remedies that everybody knows won't work," according to one government health official. One industry scientist says some doctors fear loss of control over patient treatment because "they can't control the dispensing of natural medicines by prescription." Many doctors are also understandably reluctant to recommend natural remedies about which they have little knowledge of efficacy or safety. (No pharmaceutical company representatives are knocking at their doors, giving them free samples and elaborate explanations, research results, and sales pitches to convince them to use a specific natural remedy.) It is time-consuming for practicing doctors to keep up on mainstream medications and techniques, let alone unconventional ones. Not surprisingly, many conventional doctors say they learn about natural remedies mostly from their patients.

Shaking the Snake Oil Myth

Although the idea that natural medicines are "snake oil" is fast disappearing, many still cling to it. One reason is a misunderstanding of the diverse nature of natural remedies. Plant medicine often seems foreign and unscientific to Americans because a botanical remedy does not conform to the "magic bullet" theory that a specific chemical fights only one specific disease or symptom. This theory is the foundation of the development of modern human-made pharmaceuticals. But it falls apart when one dissects the more subtle and broad therapeutic effects of plants. It is true that researchers usually identify and extract active pharmacological chemicals in plants. And natural supplements conform to standards reflecting specific proportions of those known active agents. This helps ensure that you get an active pill, but it does not totally explain why the herbal remedy, containing additional chemicals from the plant, works, or why a crude extract from the whole plant may also work. For example, one chemical in St. John's wort, hypericin, works as an antidepressant, but a broader extract of the plant works even better.

Dr. Rudi Bauer, a leading researcher on echinacea in Düsseldorf, Germany, recently spoke at a London meeting of the Society for Economic Botany on the growing scientific consensus that one constituent of a plant cannot explain its medicinal powers. More likely, he said, the improvement comes from "a synergistic effect of several diverse compounds."

Many Americans still subscribe to the doctrinaire belief that if a substance is said to treat more than one disease, it is quackery, fraud, classic "snake oil" in the tradition of worthless patent medicines that flourished in the early part of the century. That one medicine fights a single disease only has been drilled into American psyches by every well-meaning evangelistic guardian of medical establishment practice since the invention of the "magic bullet" antibiotics in the 1930s and 1940s. We still hear it and for the most part believe it. The prime hallmark of a worthless medicine, we have been told, is its multiple-purpose curative claims. It's the kiss of death for an herbal remedy in a pharmaceutically brainwashed population.

It's simply not true. Many scientifically sound reasons explain how a natural medicine can fight on many fronts at once, attacking an underlying disease process, such as inflammation, common to many diverse diseases, including arthritis, asthma, and artery disease. Feverfew, the herb that prevents migraines, is a prime example: Because of its anti-inflammatory activity, it's also used in some countries to relieve arthritis pain and respiratory problems. Even more profound are the almost universal disease-fighting powers of fish oil, which affects the functioning of every cell of every tissue and organ, and thus influences an array of diseases from the brain to the heart to the big toe.

Particularly with the exploding knowledge about the powers of antioxidants to fight disease, the "magic bullet" theory is fading into the sunset. Just the definition of an antioxidant implies divergent and broad powers of fighting disease. The theory is that out-of-control chemicals in the body called free radicals continuously attack cells, inciting virtually every chronic disease you can think of— clogged arteries, heart attacks, cancer, diabetes, cataracts, arthritis, and all the degenerative brain diseases such as Parkinson's, ALS, Huntington's, and Alzheimer's. By neutralizing these free radical thugs, antioxidants help block the appearance and progression of all such diseases.

Granted, specific types of antioxidants may be more powerful against certain disease processes, but basically they give lie to the concept that one substance treats one symptom or disease. Witness the fact that vitamin C can help ward off heart attacks and all kinds of cancers, help cure colds and relieve asthma, and probably do a lot more. The same can be said of vitamin E and one of the newer miracle medicines, coenzyme Q–10. CoQ–10 is most often used by some doctors to treat heart failure and cardiovascular disease, but its growing use against cancer is also logical. Many botanical medicines, such as ginkgo and milk thistle, are also strong antioxidants, which accounts for some of their far-flung and diverse disease-fighting activity.

Perhaps those who are stuck on the concept of the magic bullet can relate to aspirin—also of plant origin. It used to be just for pain; now it's widely touted as an anti-coagulant and anti-inflammatory agent. What does curing pain have to do with heart attacks? There is a logical underlying explanation, as there often is with many other remedies of natural origin.

Myth: Natural Drugs Misused and Unsafe

What about the assertion that conventional medicines are approved for specific uses by the Food and Drug Administration and thus are safe and effective to use, whereas natural remedies are not? It's a common fallacy that natural remedies are indiscriminately used for no valid reason, whereas conventional medicines are used only for good scientific reasons, after being tested and declared safe and effective. While it's true that the FDA must approve prescription drugs for safety and efficacy before they can be marketed, once they are approved, doctors can use them for any purpose whatever, tested or not. This is called an "off label" use of the drug, and it's pervasive. The disturbing truth is that as much as 60 percent of the drugs prescribed by doctors in this country—accounting for around a billion precriptions a year—are for "off label" uses, according to the American Medical Association; they have not been approved to treat the diseases for which they are prescribed. This means that most potent pharmaceuticals are actually being dispensed with no more proof of therapeutic efficacy than exists for natural remedies. A 1978 report by the federal Office of Technology Assessment found that only 10 to 20 percent of the treatments used by doctors had been evaluated in controlled clinical trials, the accepted standard of reliable research.

> *The practice of medicine is an art rather than a science. Most of the treatments that doctors prescribe every day are no more "proven" than the alternative methods they criticize. Accepting unproven and dangerous treatments, while rejecting safer and less expensive natural alternatives, is a bizarre double standard.*—Alan R. Gaby, M.D., as quoted in *Natural Alternatives* by Dr. Michael Murray

That natural medicines are generally unsafe is a red herring that those who are unfamiliar with botanical medicines and their track record of safety use to mislead the public. This does not mean all natural medicines are risk-free—far from it. "Natural" does not mean "benign." In fact, plants can be extremely potent, which is why they are effective in treating disease. They must be used with respect; otherwise you could harm yourself. But, generally, plant medicines have far fewer hazards than the pharmaceutical drugs many of us put in our mouths with little awareness of or concern about their possible dangerous side effects.

Thousands of Americans are harmed, even killed, by the use of such pharmaceuticals. Yet a fairly isolated case of poisoning from a natural substance, sometimes resulting from abuse, is taken as reason to condemn all over-the-counter natural remedies as hazardous to the nation's health. In two prominent national tragedies involving natural medicines, one was caused by the use of ephedra or ma huang to get high; the other was reportedly caused by toxic contaminants in l-tryptophan, properly being used as a sleeping pill. Such tragedies should not happen, and everything should be done to see they do not happen. The potential dangers and instructions for proper use of natural products should be clearly spelled out on labels, and there should be guarantees that natural remedies are free of dangerous impurities and contain what they should. This could happen through the adoption of rational regulations governing natural health products.

To be sure, what we need is a sane, solid regulatory system that will help us distinguish the effective, safe, low-cost natural medicines from the substandard stuff put out by opportunistic marketers. Most of our problems related to natural remedies could be rather quickly solved by the institution of a scientific government regulatory agency, such as the Commission E that has functioned so successfully in Germany to promote the use of natural medicines. It could be established under the National Institutes of Health and made up of both government officials and independent and industry scientists. The sooner it occurs, the better. We should no longer tolerate sloppy or fraudulent manufacturing and misleading labeling and promotion. Nor can we long afford to ignore natural medicines that are such a prominent part of sound medical practice throughout the world.

The science is here and growing. The need is here. Now is the time for all of us to start realizing the enormous potential of natural medicines by sensibly using them ourselves, and by incorporating them into our nation's medical system. What they can save us in misery and money is incalculable. And why shouldn't you be able to use these marvelous medicines with the same assurance as millions of Europeans do? Why shouldn't your doctors and your government be well informed enough to tell you about them? It is simply wrongheaded and unscientific not to acknowledge and take advantage of the vast potential benefits of these remarkable "miracle cures."

Amazing
Heart Energizer

(COENZYME Q-10)

It's a heart medicine used around the world, and if your doctor doesn't know about it, you can easily get it on your own; it could save your life.

If you have heart problems, you should know about a substance called coenzyme Q–10. It appears to be a powerful reenergizer of heart cells and can bring new hope to millions of people with heart disease, particularly those with congestive heart failure, in which heart muscle steadily weakens, causing the heart's pumping function to deteriorate. The condition is very common, especially in older people, and may not respond to conventional treatments. It stems from various causes: long-standing high blood pressure, diabetes, viral diseases, alcohol abuse, and, most frequently, a heart attack or just plain everyday damage from the aging process. Impaired, the tiny heart cells no longer generate enough energy to orchestrate the forceful heart contractions that pump blood throughout the body. Because of heart muscle cells' inefficiency, blood flow slows and heart function begins to fail. "Literally, heart failure is an energy-starved heart," says one cardiologist. Typical symptoms are shortness of breath, fatigue, fluid in the lungs, and swelling of the ankles. Gradually, the overworked heart may give out and shut down, leading to the body's steady deterioration and death. Congestive heart failure is epidemic in Western countries. It's the number one reason for hospitalization in older Americans. Common treatment: drugs such as digitalis, diuretics, vasodilators, and ACE inhibitors. The ultimate cure: heart transplant. But there's another common treatment that's used throughout the world with great success. It reenergizes the heart by giving cells a renewed burst of energy. It's called coenzyme Q–10, and its miracles are legendary among some cardiologists.

SUSAN'S MIRACLE
From Death's Door to Recovery

In October 1994 Susan Porter* appeared to be dying of heart failure. "She was miserable, so weak she could barely sit up," says her daughter Joan. "Mom couldn't breathe, was fatigued, and had a lot of swelling in her lungs. We canceled my parents' fiftieth wedding anniversary party because Mom was too weak to go, even in a wheelchair. She was ready to throw in the towel, and her doctors had basically given up. She was too old for heart transplant. She had been treated with all the traditional medicine and she was not getting any better. We didn't think she would make it to Thanksgiving."

After years of high blood pressure, Mrs. Porter had been diagnosed with congestive heart failure nineteen years earlier. With drugs, including ACE inhibitors (Capoten) and increasing doses of diuretics, she had lived a very active life—until the last six months, when her condition had progressively deteriorated to the life-threatening stage. When Dr. Stephen T. Sinatra, a board-certified internist and cardiologist at Manchester (Connecticut) Memorial Hospital, reviewed her case, he agreed she was in severe congestive heart failure. "She was absolutely a wreck, suffering from end stage cardiac cachexia —severe weakness and weight loss," he says. At age seventy-nine, Mrs. Porter weighed only 77 pounds; her heart's "ejection fraction"—a measure of its pumping ability—had fallen to a mere 10 to 15 percent (normal is 50 to 70 percent), meaning that little blood and oxygen were getting to her vital organs. "Her heart barely pumped enough to support her bed-to-chair existence," recalls Dr. Sinatra. He suggested that, in addition to her other standard medications, Susan start taking 30 milligrams of coenzyme Q–10 three times a day, a dose Dr. Sinatra had found effective in other cardiac patients. But it didn't help much, and Susan continued to go downhill. In February 1995 she was near death; fluid had built up in her lungs and abdomen; she breathed with great difficulty. The signs were very bad that her body was shutting down.

Then in March 1995 the most remarkable, fortuitous mistake occurred. "Her son caused the miracle," says Dr. Sinatra. Instead of picking up a bottle of 30-milligram coQ–10 capsules at the health food store, her son Steve accidentally picked up a bottle of 100-milligram coQ–10 capsules. She was now taking 300 milligrams of coQ–10 a day by mistake—more than triple her usual dose. One month later, in April, she had improved so dramatically on coQ–10 that she got up and went to her son's house for Easter dinner. "We could hardly believe it," says her daughter. "Her energy was back. The swelling in her legs was going down, the fluid in her lungs was gone. The coQ–10 was working." She continued to improve, and by June her heart's ejection fraction was up to 20 percent. That may not sound like a lot, but when it is so low, 5 percent can make a big difference, says Dr. Sinatra. There was also markedly less "mitral and tricuspid regurgitation"—leakage and backflow of blood into the heart's upper chambers. This made the heart's pumping more efficient and lessened fluid buildup in tissue.

By October Susan was out shopping; in November she started going to church again; in December she traveled to visit her daughter for the first time in a year and a half. In January she was walking to the car when she missed a step and fractured her hip; her heart was strong enough to survive total hip replacement. She recovered to the point of walking without a cane. Although Susan has developed troubling thyroid problems unrelated to her heart failure, "she is peppy and has not been readmitted to the hospital for her heart since she started taking coQ–10," said her daughter in February 1997. Her son refers to his mother as "the lady with nine lives." She continues to take 300 milligrams of coQ–10 every day.

*A pseudonym has been used to protect privacy but the medical details are correct.

What Is It?

Coenzyme Q-10 is a strong antioxidant known also as ubiquinol–10. It has been described as "vitaminlike," but some experts say it is a definitely a vitamin—that is, a nutrient your body must take in to feed your cells so your body can operate at an optimum level. It is present in very small amounts in food, notably seafood, and is produced by all cells of the body. Japanese scientists have synthesized coQ–10 into a raw material that is put into supplements and sold throughout the world by several Japanese companies.

What's the Evidence?

Compelling evidence shows that most heart patients are deficient in coQ–10 and that taking coQ–10 supplements revitalizes heart function and can dramatically relieve heart disease symptoms. Pioneering studies by Karl Folkers, Ph.D., director of the Institute for Biomedical Research at the University of Texas at Austin, showed that 75 percent of heart patients have severe deficiencies of coQ–10 in heart tissue compared with healthy individuals. Further, he documented that taking coenzyme Q–10 significantly benefited three-fourths of a group of elderly patients with congestive heart failure. More than fifty major articles have been published in reputable medical journals worldwide in the last ten years on the use of coQ–10 for heart disease, primarily congestive heart failure.

Extensive Japanese research has found that about 70 percent of patients improved on coQ–10. CoQ–10 is also widely used in Italy, having been tested in trials at several centers involving 2,500 patients. Eighty percent of heart-failure patients improved after taking 100 milligrams of coQ–10 along with conventional therapy. In a follow-up study, 50 milligrams of coQ–10 daily for a month, alone or with other treatments, significantly improved symptoms of heart failure and quality of life. Because of the international research on coQ–10, it is a drug of choice in many countries. It is "routinely" given to patients with congestive heart failure in Israeli hospitals. Japanese doctors have used coQ–10 for cardiac problems for more than thirty years. It is now among the top six pharmaceutical agents used in Japan. If you have heart failure in Italy, it's likely to be recommended.

Dr. Sinatra, who is also an assistant clinical professor at the University of Connecticut School of Medicine, is one of a growing number of American physicians using coQ–10. "I personally use Q–10 for every one of my patients with congestive heart failure if they are willing to take it," he says. He has treated thousands of heart patients with coQ–10, and he estimates it has helped more than 70 percent of them. Some of his failures, he believes, were due to doses that were inadequate or products without sufficient potency. The dose must be enough to substantially raise blood levels of coQ–10; if that happens, he believes, about 100 percent of heart patients would benefit.

EXCITING NEW RESEARCH IN CANADA
The Case of the Unneeded Pacemaker

At last, coenzyme Q–10 is due to get some massive mainstream attention, thanks to Dr. Michael Sole, a professor of medicine at the University of Toronto and director of the Peter Munk Cardiac Centre, one of the world's largest and most prominent centers for the treatment and study of heart disease. It's time, says Dr. Sole, to seriously investigate the potential of using coQ–10 to treat heart disease, particularly heart failure, on the basis of the enormous amount of data, including studies by Dr. Karl Folkers, already in the medical literature. Dr.

Sole and colleagues are beginning animal studies with coQ–10, to be followed by studies on humans with heart disease, primarily heart failure. The researchers at first will look mainly at coQ–10's effects on heart function and metabolic changes in the heart for a period of three to six months. (The patients will continue to take their regular heart medications.)

Dr. Sole confesses that his interest was piqued by an experience with a patient who needed a pacemaker, didn't get one, but recovered anyway. "I had this patient with a deteriorating heart condition who developed a heart block and needed a pacemaker," says Dr. Sole. "I referred him to get one implanted, but when I saw him four months later, he hadn't had his pacemaker put in. To my surprise, his condition, which had been deteriorating over the last several years, had remarkably reversed itself. So I said to him, 'Wow, this is amazing! I've never seen anything like this in my entire experience as a cardiologist.' At which point the patient confessed to me he didn't want a pacemaker and after seeing me had talked to a friend who was taking coenzyme Q–10, so he decided to take it himself." Was the coQ–10 responsible or coincidental in this startling case? As Dr. Sole says, it is merely one case, and he doesn't know the answer. "But it was dramatic enough to make me wonder. Of course, I've seen miracles come and go, and whether coQ–10 is one is something we need to explore by doing the type of double-blind controlled studies that will tell us for sure. At the moment, it sure looks promising enough to be worthy of our further investigation."

How Does It Work?

CoQ–10 is a unique antioxidant that reportedly penetrates the cells' tiny "energy factories," called mitochondria, where oxygen is burned, giving cells energy to carry on the business of life. To efficiently burn energy, the mitochondria need coQ–10. It is often called the "spark" that starts and helps drive the mitochondrial engines.

Without enough coQ–10, the theory goes, cells suffer power shortages, impairing the function of vital organs, most noticeably the heart, which needs the most coQ–10 to generate the tremendous energy needed to keep the heart beating. When damaged heart muscle cells are depleted of vital coQ–10, energy production is low, resulting in mitochondrial and cardiovascular dysfunction. Supplying the heart muscle with coQ–10 supplements revitalizes energy-starved cells, boosting power output, leading to a more efficient heart that doesn't have to work so hard to circulate blood, say experts. In short, coQ–10 improves mechanical function of the heart by giving energy-starved cells the fuel needed to function efficiently. CoQ–10 may also help prevent and heal degenerative damage to heart cells and help keep "bad" LDL cholesterolfrom clogging arteries.

How Much Do You Need?

A typical dose for heart disease is 50 to 150 milligrams a day; however, up to 300 milligrams a day may be needed when heart failure is severe. Dr. Sinatra says that the sicker the cardiac patient, the weaker the heart, the higher the coQ–10 dose needs to be. Some researchers recommend 2 milligrams of coQ–10 for each kilogram (2.2 pounds) of body weight. Critically important is the fact that, to be effective, the dose of coQ–10 must significantly raise blood levels of coQ–10. The amount needed to do that varies among individuals, and also depends on the potency or "bioavailability" of the coQ–10 used. Some people get a good rise with 100 milligrams, whereas others need two or three times that much to attain the same blood level, says internationally-known cardiologist-researcher Peter H. Langsjoen in Bullard, Texas, who uses coQ–10 extensively in his practice and has done research with Dr. Folkers.

The only way to be sure if coQ–10 is working and to determine what dose is needed is to measure blood levels, he says.

How Quickly Does It Work?
Typically, it takes two to eight weeks for coQ–10 to produce an improvement in symptoms of heart failure, say authorities. You must take coQ–10 continually to maintain its heart-strengthening benefits. It is not a permanent, short-time cure.

The Safety Factor
Side effects are minor and rare, usually nothing more than mild transient nausea. In the large Italian study, 22 out of 2,664 patients reported mild side effects, or slightly less than 1 percent. No toxicity has been found, even at high doses, in animals or humans, says Dr. Folkers.

Caution: Remember that coQ–10 is not a substitute for conventional drugs, but is usually used along with conventional therapy for best results. CoQ–10 may allow you to reduce dosage of conventional drugs, but you should do this with the supervision of your doctor. Although many people with varying degrees of atherosclerosis, which virtually all adults have by middle age, may want to take coQ–10 as a preventive, heart failure is a serious condition that should not be self-diagnosed or self-medicated. If you have serious heart disease, always consult a doctor for the proper course of treatment.

Consumer Concerns

All coQ-10 is made in Japan and sold to numerous companies that package it in pressed tablets, powder-filled capsules, or gel caps. Because coQ-10 is fat-soluble, it's essential to take dry coQ-10 with some fat for absorption. If you simply gulp down a dry coQ-10 tablet, much of it is wasted. One cardiologist suggests taking it with a little peanut butter or olive oil. New research, however, shows that coQ-10 in soft gel capsules is often superior to the dry form; the soft gel's coQ-10 bioavailability—how much gets into your bloodstream—can be several times greater than that of coQ-10 dry tablets or capsules, according to recent tests. That means that certain soft gels are much more potent; thus, you need to take fewer of them to get the same blood-level boost of coQ-10. Two soft gel makers that claim three to four times higher bioavailability than that of dry coQ-10 pills are Soft Gel Technologies in Los Angeles, California (800-360-7484) and the Tishcon Corp. in Westbury, N.Y. (800-848-8442). Their soft gels are sold under many different brand names, too numerous to list here.

You can also get chewable coQ-10 pills that have far higher bioavailability than plain dry powdered tablets you swallow, says Dr. Langsjoen. A chewable wafer he uses personally and has been used in research studies is available from the Vitaline Corp. in Ashland, Oregon (800-648-4755). Unfortunately, coQ-10, partly because of the Japanese monopoly, is relatively costly.

What Else Is It Good For?

Coenzyme Q-10's main claim to fame is relieving congestive heart failure. However, studies show it is also successful in treating other forms of cardiovascular problems: high blood pressure, arrhythmia (irregular heartbeats), angina (chest pain), and mitral valve prolapse. Because of its strong antioxidant properties, coQ–10 is also being tested in patients with degenerative neurological diseases, Parkinson's disease, Huntington's disease, ALS (amyotrophic lateral sclerosis) and multiple sclerosis at major medical centers, including the University of Rochester Medical School and the University of California at San Diego. The hope is that coQ–10 can slow down progression of the diseases.

CANCER: THE NEXT FRONTIER?
Coenzyme Q–10 is also being studied to treat cancer, notably breast cancer, with some reported dramatic successes. Texas researcher Dr. Folkers, the man who pioneered the use of coQ–10 in heart failure, has now documented that cancer patients, too, often have deficiencies of coQ–10. Recently Dr. Folkers reported that six of ten Americans became free of cancer during therapy with coQ–10 and survived five to fifteen years. Much research on cancer patients, inspired by Dr. Folkers, has been done in Copenhagen by Danish cancer specialist Knut Lockwood. He uses high doses of various antioxidants, including coQ–10, and fatty acids as an adjunct to conventional breast cancer therapy, including a combination of surgery, chemotherapy, radiotherapy, and drugs such as tamoxifen, as routinely demanded in Denmark.

TWO DANISH WOMEN'S MIRACLES
"The Cancers Just Disappeared"

In 1992 Danish researcher Knut Lockwood at his Copenhagen cancer clinic began testing coQ–10 and other antioxidants on thirty-two breast cancer patients, ages thirty-two to eighty-one. His study is ongoing, and he expects to report long-term results in 1998. In the interim, Dr. Lockwood and colleagues, including Dr. Karl Folkers at the University of Texas, have published several astonishing cases of remission in women with metastasized breast cancer who have used the supplements along with conventional therapies. Here are two cases published in *Biochemical and Biophysical Research Communications* and *Molecular Aspects of Medicine* in 1994 and 1995.

Amazing Regression In July 1991 at age fifty-nine, K.M. had surgery for breast cancer. In October she entered Dr. Lockwood's study and started taking a large number of daily supplements as called for in his protocol, including 2,850 milligrams of vitamin C; 2,500 international units (IU) of vitamin E; 32.5 IU of beta-carotene; 387 micrograms of selenium, 1.2 grams of gamma linolenic acid (GLA), 3.5 grams of omega–3 fatty acids (fish oil), and 90 milligrams of coenzyme Q–10. The cancer did not metastasize outside the breast, but a cancer did reappear in the breast. Close observation by mammogram showed that the tumor was not growing. Indeed, for about a year it seemingly "stabilized at 1.5 to 2 centimeters."

In October 1993 Dr. Lockwood and colleagues decided to raise the patient's dose of coQ–10 to 390 milligrams a day. One month later, to the doctors' surprise, they could no longer "palpate," or feel the tumor by touch. By December the cancer had disappeared from the mammogram; there were no traces of a mass or any signs of microcalcifications on the X-ray. The cancer was in complete regression—

gone! Dr. Lockwood, who has treated more than 200 cases of breast cancer per year for thirty-five years, said he had never before witnessed a spontaneous complete regression of a breast tumor measuring as much as 1.5 to 2 centimeters. Further, he had never seen a comparable regression from any conventional antitumor therapy.

Deadly Cancer Gone In September 1992 a forty-four-year-old woman patient of Dr. Lockwood's had a double mastectomy, the surgical removal of both breasts after discovery of cancer. The cancer had already spread to two out of twelve lymph nodes in the right armpit. She received a series of ten treatments of chemotherapy.

In April 1994 tests revealed that the breast cancer had metastasized to her liver. So serious is this that in the words of her doctors, "Metastases in the liver can be regarded as a prelude to imminent death."

Her dose of coQ–10 was also raised from 90 milligrams to 390 milligrams a day. She continued to take the usual regimen of supplements she had been on since the double mastectomy, along with 30 milligrams of tamoxifen daily. In April 1995 a liver echoscan showed that the cancerous cells in her liver had totally disappeared. Nor were there any signs of cancer spread to any other part of her body.

Dr. Lockwood credited the coenzyme Q–10 for the regression of the breast cancer and remission of the liver cancer, saying such occurrences from conventional treatment alone are extremely rare. He thinks most breast cancer patients should be given coQ-10 along with conventional therapy. The daily dose: between 90 and 390 milligrams for the average patient, he says.

Note: Coenzyme Q–10 is a very powerful antioxidant that does have anticancer activity in test tube and animal studies, and some doctors add coQ–10 to vitamin-dietary supplements given to cancer patients in the United States. Although no one can really know what causes a "spontaneous remission" of any cancer, these cases have medical plausibility for anticancer action by coQ–10. Note that coQ–10 was not used alone but was given with other agents, including standard cancer drugs, and that Drs. Lockwood and Folkers do recommend coQ–10 not as a magic bullet, but as an adjunct to conventional cancer therapy, an added agent to help push cancer into remission.

The Prozac of Plants

(ST. JOHN'S WORT—HYPERICUM)

In Germany the number one drug for depression is not Prozac; it's nature's own version of Prozac. You can easily get it here, too, if you need it.

If you suffer from mild to moderate depression, before you opt for the heavy brain artillery of strong antidepressants with hazardous side effects and a hefty price tag, you may want to consider a remedy successfully used and extensively tested in Europe—a plant extract called St. John's wort, or hypericum. It's the drug of choice for common depression in Germany, where it outsells all other antidepressants combined and outsells Prozac by more than seven to one. Every year German doctors write about 3 million prescriptions for St. John's wort, based on government approval and the results of stringent clinical tests. Around twenty-five meticulously conducted studies find that the herb relieves depression often as effectively as strong antidepressant drugs, and without unpleasant side effects.

At long last American doctors and government officials are becoming excited about St. John's wort as a benign but potent treatment for some forms of depression. The European evidence is so impressive that the National

Institute of Mental Health is launching a groundbreaking clinical study to see whether hypericum, as it is called medically, can be sanctioned by health officials as an alternative to current antidepressants. If it proves to work better than a placebo (inactive pill) and perhaps as well as or better than prescription drugs, such as Prozac, it will be a blessing for millions of Americans who need antidepressants but fear the potentially alarming side effects, says Dr. Jerry Cott, chief of research on pharmacologic treatment at NIMH. But the good news is that you don't have to wait to try it, because it is already available as a "dietary supplement" without FDA approval. It has already helped millions of Europeans and Americans.

ELIZABETH'S MIRACLE CURE
"I Was Really Depressed and It Gave Me My Life Back"

It was one of those bizarre events you never think will happen. In 1985 Elizabeth Dante, a young mother in Laguna Hills, California, contracted polio from a polio vaccine. She was paralyzed for a year, was told she would never walk again, and suffered a constant burning pain in her neck and legs. Not surprisingly, she became dependent on a daily regimen of painkillers. By 1992 she realized she was severely depressed, even suicidal. She and her husband were alarmed. "It got increasingly difficult for me to function on a daily basis. I've had depressions where it scared me. It was dark, really dark," she recalls.

Then four years ago her husband gave her a book entitled *How to Heal Depression*, by Harold

Bloomfield, M.D., a psychiatrist in Del Mar, California. Impressed, she went to him. He prescribed one antidepressant, then another, but both had to be discontinued because of disagreeable side effects. Dr. Bloomfield then prescribed Paxil, a popular antidepressant, a cousin to Prozac. It did the trick. She felt better, more energetic, though perhaps a little bit "drugged," and she took the drug religiously because "I never wanted to feel those scary suicidal moments again."

After about three years, she wanted to get off Paxil. "Because of the history I had with painkillers I didn't want to get hooked on anything. I just wanted to be drug-free." But it was risky. Dr. Bloomfield had a suggestion: a natural antidepressant, widely used in Germany, called St. John's wort, or hypericum. "I was a little skeptical, but I thought, Hey, I'm going to try this." She also knew that if the old feelings of depression returned, she could go back on Paxil. Dr. Bloomfield gave her a schedule to follow in which she gradually reduced the dose of Paxil and increased the dose of St. John's wort. After a few weeks she was entirely off Paxil and feeling better than she had felt in years. "I could feel the effect of the St. John's wort even faster than Dr. Bloomfield said I would. It was a smooth transition.

"I feel tremendously normal. It sounds so ordinary, but when you've had a history of chronic pain and depression, to feel normal is like feeling high! It's a wonderful feeling. I don't feel drugged; I feel very healthy. I wake up in the morning with a smile on my face, which has not happened in years and years and years, even on the Paxil. It's like my old personality from a long time ago is here again." She is also off painkillers. With the help of therapy, she has learned to walk and even dance a little. Dante continues to take a capsule of St. John's wort three times a day, paying about 8 cents a pill. Paxil, she says, cost around $2 a pill.

She can hardly say enough for St. John's wort. "It's fabulous. I like it a lot. I would recommend it to anyone! It's really given me my life back in many ways."

JOEL'S MIRACLE
"It Worked When Other Drugs Failed"

Now age forty-three, Joel Rutledge, M.D.,* has suffered a lifetime of depression, receiving psychological counseling in his teens and antidepressants in his twenties. For the most part the antidepressants kept his depression under control. But the drugs often had to be changed to control his illness. And in the winter of 1996 the effectiveness of his current antidepressants was fading. He was stricken with feelings of intense sadness, worthlessness, apathy, overwhelming fatigue, and loss of energy. He took little pleasure in his work as a physician or in life in general.

His diagnosis is serious "double depression"— major depression with a component of seasonal affective disorder or SAD, also called the "winter blues," in which changes in brain chemistry caused by deprivation of sunlight bring on dark moods. Joel was under the care of Dr. Norman Rosenthal, who is an authority on SAD and a researcher at the National Institute of Mental Health. Dr. Rosenthal is knowledgeable about European research on St. John's wort and thought the botanical medicine might help Joel overcome his worsening depression. In January Joel started taking hypericum (the medical term) in doses of 300-milligram pills three times a day. This was in addition to his other prescription drugs, artificial light therapy, and psychiatric counseling. Such multifaceted therapy is common in depression, and prescription antidepressants are often combined for maximum benefit. Finding the right drug to add when others fail is tricky, but if it succeeds, it can have a dramatic impact.

That's what happened when Joel took St. John's wort. The benefit was unexpectedly swift and striking. After only a couple of doses, Joel says, his mood lightened and his energy returned. "Within a week or two, he felt a big difference. It was very quick," agrees Dr. Rosenthal. So remarkable was St. John's wort that Joel continues to take it enthusiastically, and Dr. Rosenthal has suggested it to other patients with success. He plans further investigations and is excited by the possibility that St. John's wort might be used as adjunct treatment for many others who are not fully responding to their medications. "It's good stuff," in Dr. Rosenthal's view. After all, Joel's depression had persisted, despite all the conventional antidepressants. Yet an herbal remedy was able to step in and work side by side with established antidepressants to lift Joel out of his lethargy and dark moods. "That's extremely impressive," says Dr. Rosenthal.

*A pseudonym has been used to protect privacy, but the medical details are accurate.

What Is It?

Scientifically known as *Hypericum perforatum*, St. John's wort is a common wildflower with vivid yellow flowers edged with tiny black beads. When rubbed, the plant releases a red pigment, containing hypericin, identified as a pharmacologically active chemical. The name comes from Christian folklore; the plant's red spots are said to symbolize the blood spilled by St. John the Baptist when he was beheaded. The plant blooms around June 24 in Germany, the traditional birthday of John the Baptist. "Wort" means "plant" in Old English.

What's the Evidence?

St. John's wort as an antidepressant for treating mild to moderate depression has been confirmed by numerous well designed studies comparing the herb with both inactive "sugar " pills (placebos) and other antidepressants. Most of the recent research has been done in Germany and Austria, using a St. John's wort formula, known as LI 160, which is widely sold as a drug. Rigorous studies show that about 60 to 80 percent of depressed individuals improve on St. John's wort, which is about the same as that expected from conventional synthetic antidepressants. In a recent German survey of 3,250 depressed patients and their physicians, 80 percent reported improvement or freedom from symptoms after taking St. John's wort for four weeks.

There's no question that St. John's wort works, as a string of studies show. One study of 105 persons with depression, by researchers at the University of Salzburg, found that St. John's wort was 250 percent better than a placebo. Sixty-seven percent of subjects taking 900 milligrams of St. John's wort daily improved dramatically within four weeks, compared with 28 percent on placebo. The botanical antidepressant improved mood, emotional fear, and psychosomatic symptoms, such as disturbed sleep, headache, cardiac troubles, and exhaustion.

A similar study of thirty-nine patients found that 70 percent were depression-free after a month. Symptoms best treated: lack of activity, tiredness, fatigue, sleep disturbances. Another major German study of 135 depressed patients at several medical centers compared 900 milligrams daily of St. John's wort with 75 milligrams of imipramine, a popular tricyclic antidepressant. The herb scored as well as—on some measurements even 25 percent better than—the manmade pharmaceutical, and was far safer, producing fewer and milder side effects. Other research declared St. John's wort equal to or even better than the drug maprotiline in fighting depression and improving cognitive (thinking) functions, as confirmed by EEG brain tracings.

St. John's wort also can relieve seasonal affective disorder (SAD)—the "winter blues," a common mood disorder due to sunlight deprivation. The usual treatment is light therapy. But St. John's wort also fights the depression, according to Dr. Siegfried Kasper, of the University of Vienna, Austria, and Begona Martinez of the Psychiatric University Clinic in Bonn, Germany. They gave SAD patients 900 milligrams of St. John's wort (called extract LI 160) daily and judged it so effective that they considered it an alternative to light therapy. However, the herbal medicine was even more potent taken along with light therapy.

Summing up the evidence for St. John's wort's effectiveness as an antidepressant is an evaluation of twenty-three randomized clinical trials with 1,757 patients, published in the prestigious *British Medical Journal* in 1996. Researchers Gilbert Ramirez, of the University of North Texas Health Science Center in Fort Worth, and Klaus Linde, of Munich's Ludwig-Maximilians-Universität, applied the same stringent standards of scientific proof to St. John's wort and to orthodox pharmaceutical antidepressants. Their conclusion: St. John's wort equals conventional antidepressants in efficacy. In other words, St. John's wort is just as apt to relieve commonplace depression as a prescription antidepressant. Critically important: St. John's wort, unlike prescription drugs, is relatively free of unwanted side effects.

The two doctors searched the medical literature for every valid study on St. John's wort. Interestingly, they said that if they had confined their search to studies published in English, they would have found none. Most were in German, and thus denied to most American, British, and other English-speaking doctors—and, consequently, to their patients.

In Germany St. John's wort is approved as a treatment for mild to moderate depression, anxiety and nervous unrest.

How Does It Work?

Theoretically St. John's wort may work on many systems of the brain simultaneously through different chemical constituents. "At this moment nobody really knows exactly how the plant works to relieve depression," says psychopharmacologist Jerry Cott of the National Institute of Mental Health, although research shows the plant extract has activity similar to that of certain prescription antidepressants. At first scientists believed that St. John's wort worked like so-called MAO-inhibitor antidepressants, such as Nardil, that block the enzyme monoaminooxidase from destroying two important "feel good" brain chemicals, serotonin and norepinephrine. But new evidence shows that St. John's wort is not an MAO-inhibitor except at extremely high doses, about 100 times those recommended to treat depression. New research suggests that St John's wort actually relieves depression by acting as a "serotonin reuptake inhibitor," which is the way Prozac works.

However, which specific chemicals in St. John's wort account for its antidepressant activity is unclear, says Dr. Cott. Long identified as the most likely candidate is hypericin, the plant's red pigment and a documented psychotropic agent. But recent research finds hypericin less potent an antidepressant than the whole plant extract itself, suggesting the herb's complex mixture of chemicals, including xanthones and flavonoids, also are critical in the plant's pharmacological benefits.

How Much Do You Need?
The recommended adult dose for mild to moderate depression, as determined in studies, is one tablet or capsule of 300 milligrams of St. John's wort extract (standardized to contain 0.3 percent of hypericin), taken three times a day. That supplies a daily dose of about 1 milligram of hypericin, one of the extract's primary active ingredients. Check the label to be sure the product is "standardized" for the right amount of hypericin.

New research by Dr. E. U. Vorbach at the Clinic for Psychiatry and Psychotherapy in Darmstadt, Germany, also finds that higher doses of St. John's wort—1,800 milligrams daily, which is double the typical dose—can relieve *severe* depression, as long as the patient has no psychotic or delusional symptoms. His research found no increased side effects from the higher doses.

How Quickly Does It Work?
Although a few people have seen relief rather quickly, within two weeks, typically it takes several weeks. One

study found that more than half the benefits from taking St. John's wort came between four and eight weeks. Animal studies also suggest that hypericum and its antidepressive effects accumulate in the brain. Give the natural medicine at least six weeks to work, urge some experts.

What Can You Expect?

St. John's wort may not work for everyone or as well as prescription antidepressants for some. But, on the basis of studies, it appears that a remarkable 80 percent of those taking it will feel better. On some mood evaluation tests, 70 to 90 percent of patients on St. John's wort have improved, compared with 42 percent to 55 percent on placebo. One analysis of 3,250 patients found that only 15 percent had no response.

The Safety Factor

One of the most attractive features of St. John's wort is that its side effects are rare and relatively benign, says Dr. Michael A. Jenike in an editorial in the *Journal of Geriatric Psychiatry and Neurology*. The complaint most often reported is gastrointestinal upset. Allergies to St. John's wort are unusual. All side effects reportedly go away quickly when you stop taking the herb; no permanent harm has been reported. In studies, mild reversible side effects from St. John's wort have ranged from less than 1 percent to 10 percent. That's compared with 36 percent of prescription antidepressant users who sometimes suffer extremely serious and lasting harm. Sometimes lowering the dose slightly to let your body adapt to the herbal medicine makes side effects disappear.

Some doctors warn hypericum users to stay out of the sun, because of "photosensitive" poisoning or skin reactions. That has happened in light-skinned animals grazing on St. John's wort, but it would take about thirty to seventy times the recommended antidepressant doses to cause such problems in humans, studies indicate. The extensive use of the herbal remedy in Germany has not produced evidence of short-term or long-term toxicity at recommended therapeutic doses.

People who are on other antidepressants or have severe depression, psychotic symptoms, and suicidal thoughts should take St. John's wort only with the advice and supervision of a doctor. Depression can be a serious illness, and self-diagnosing and self-medicating to treat it is risky. Also, don't take St. John's wort if you are pregnant or lactating. Nor should it be given to children, except on a physician's advice. Don't take it in combination with prescription antidepressants, except under medical supervision.

What's the Alternative?

Generally, mild to moderate depression is treated with several methods of psychotherapy, including cognitive behavioral therapy, light therapy, sleep modification, and, mainly, prescription antidepressant drugs. About forty such pharmaceutical antidepressants are on the market. The main concern with all of them is the potential for serious adverse reactions, affecting mainly the nervous system, but also the cardiovascular system.

IF YOU WANT TO TRY ST. JOHN'S WORT

Here's advice from Dr. Norman Rosenthal, a research psychiatrist at the National Institute of Mental Health and an international authority on depression. Dr. Rosenthal urges everyone to use St.

John's wort only with medical supervision, because self-treating depression can be hazardous. However, since many physicians and other health professionals are not yet knowledgeable about St. John's wort, he offers these guidelines:

- Do not count on St. John's wort as a magic bullet to cure depression. It is most effective used with other therapies, including counseling and sometimes other medications.
- If you are taking prescription antidepressants, don't quit suddenly and substitute St. John's wort. A quick withdrawal from prescription antidepressants could cause a "rebound" effect with potentially serious consequences.
- To get off antidepressants, such as Prozac and Paxil, slowly reduce the doses while gradually introducing St. John's wort.
- St. John's wort is best recommended for treating mild to moderate depression, since most of the research has been done on patients with such depression. Increasing evidence suggests the herb can also relieve some types of severe depression (not manic depression), but the research is not as extensive or firm in such cases.
- Take St. John's wort for at least six weeks before deciding whether it works. Quitting any earlier is too soon, since, as with other antidepressants, it will take a while for St. John's wort to produce benefits.
- If your depression worsens or you have suicidal impulses, or you notice severe side effects while taking St. John's wort, stop taking it and see your doctor immediately. Mild side effects tend to dis-

appear as your body adapts to the medication; if not, consult a health professional.

Consumer Concerns

To be sure you get a consistent, measurable dose of the active material every time, you need a standardized high-quality product. In Germany the most thoroughly tested and most widely sold St. John's wort pill—accounting for 200,000 prescriptions per month compared with 30,000 for Prozac—is a chemical formula known as LI 160 and sold under the brand name Jarsin. You can now get the identical research-grade St. John's wort formula in the United States under the brand name Kira, which is made by Lichtwer Pharma of Berlin. Kira was recently introduced in Wal-Mart stores and is scheduled to be widely available in similar retail outlets and health food stores later in the year. Expected retail price: $15 for a bottle of forty-five 300-milligram tablets.

Consumers can also check the website of California psychiatrist Harold H. Bloomfield, an authority on St. John's wort and author of the book *Hypericum & Depression*, for updates on St. John's wort products and research. The website is http://www.hypericum.com.

Astonishing Memory Pill

(GINKGO)

It's a potent brain medicine that can save your failing memory, if you take it early enough. Don't wait until it's too late.

When memory seems less sharp, or other signs of impending mental decline set in with age, most people feel helpless and hopeless, caught in humanity's fateful "seventh age"—that relentless march toward "senility" that presumably cannot be halted. The gradual diminution of memory and mental faculties, known medically as dementia, is usually passed off as the cruel and inevitable consequences of getting old. Is it true? Is there nothing to take, no drug, no pill that might retard the pace of mental deterioration as we age? Are we truly absolute victims of brain cell degeneration that may render us mentally incompetent or put us deep into the oblivion of Alzheimer's disease?

To say that a substance to treat failing mental faculties exists in the leaf of a common tree may seem incredible. Yet such a plant medicine is used throughout Europe and the Far East as a potion of considerable ancient and modern reputation for treating age-related decline in mental functions. Its use is slowly but surely making its way into the offices of doctors and the highest scientific circles in this country. It is called ginkgo biloba, and its beneficial effects on blood circulation and brain function make this herb a remarkable medicine. It works in both neurodegenerative and vascular diseases, such as poor blood flow to the brain because of narrowed blood vessels—a common cause of impaired memory and other symptoms of so-called "senility." In Germany and France ginkgo is widely prescribed as a treatment for age-related mental malfunction, including general dementia and Alzheimer's. And the scientific evidence for its efficacy and safety is extensive and compelling, especially when it is pitted against the paucity of conventional alternatives; drugs approved for memory loss and Alzheimer's in the United States are of limited effectiveness and fraught with serious side effects.

Ginkgo can work wonders in the brain to halt brain deterioration, postponing the onset of "senility" and perhaps even rejuvenating some mental faculties, with a very minor risk of side effects. The astonishing fact is that we all have easy access to a simple plant medicine that impeccable research shows can help protect the most important organ in our body, our brain, the source of our humanity and personality, from deteriorating as we get older and creating major personal and societal misery. Yet very few Americans, outside research circles, have ever heard of it.

DR. JERRY COTT'S MIRACLE
"Ginkgo Stopped My Mother's Decline"

Dr. Jerry Cott, a psychopharmacologist and chief of the Pharmacologic Treatment Research Program at the National Institute of Mental Health, has studied the pharmacological activity of ginkgo in brain cells and is familiar with the large body of European scientific evidence supporting its effectiveness. He is convinced it helps retard the loss of memory and mental capabilities due to "mini strokes" and even Alzheimer's disease. In fact, his own mother, Eula Cott, began to have memory problems when she was in her late seventies. Four years later, she was diagnosed with Alzheimer's disease. She went to the NIMH clinical center in Bethesda, Maryland, for experimental treatment with various drugs. None worked, and after six months she was released back to her family.

Her scientist son began giving her ginkgo biloba in standardized doses of 240 milligrams daily, which is used in Germany to treat Alzheimer's. She did not suddenly recover her lost memory, because you wouldn't expect ginkgo to revive dead brain cells, says Dr. Cott. But something extraordinary did happen. Her Alzheimer's has not progressed as it would invariably be expected to do. "Definitely, you would normally see a measurable deterioration every six months. But she has not gotten a smidgen worse in four years, which I think is pretty remarkable, and so do her other doctors," says Dr. Cott. He thinks that is the real promise of ginkgo, that it can intervene in the progressive damage to brain cells, thus halting or dramatically slowing down the worsening memory loss and other signs of one of our most heartbreaking disorders, for which there is no other real treatment. "I would never give my mother tacrine [an FDA drug approved for Alzheimer's] because the side effects are too awful, and similar drugs had not worked," says Dr. Cott.

But ginkgo is virtually benign. Her son is convinced it has helped his mother, now age eighty-eight, function with dignity in an assisted-living center far better and longer than would have been expected otherwise.

What Is It?
The medicine called ginkgo biloba is derived from the leaves of the ginkgo tree, an ornamental tree growing in temperate climates. The plant's reputed most active chemicals, the ginkgolides, are generally extracted from the leaves and turned into tablets of various potency. These potent ginkgolides are unique to the ginkgo tree and are not found anywhere else in nature.

What's the Evidence?
Some experts call ginkgo the most important of all botanical medicines. Since the 1950s more than 400 papers on ginkgo, most from German investigators, have appeared in the medical literature. More than fifty controlled clinical trials confirm ginkgo biloba as a treatment for diminished memory and concentration, increased absentmindedness, confusion, energy loss, tiredness, depression, dizziness, and tinnitus (ringing in the ears.) Specifically, researchers have documented the use of ginkgo in treating dementia, including Alzheimer's.

The impact of ginkgo can be enormous, revitalizing brain activity and stopping or reversing a constellation of symptoms due to poor blood flow. According to one German study, blood flow increased 57 percent one hour after ginkgo was taken, as measured in subjects' capillaries. Two other recent well-conducted German studies showed impressive effects after regular use of ginkgo. One found that ginkgo improved brain function by a striking 72 percent on average after three months of use by ninety-nine older patients who had suffered brain disturbances for about two years. In another study of 200 patients, average age sixty-nine, who had endured memory problems for about four years, 71 percent improved after three months on ginkgo, compared with 32 percent on placebo.

A compelling endorsement of ginkgo came from Drs. Jos Kleijnen and Paul Knipschild at the University of Limburg in Maastricht, the Netherlands. In 1992, as reported in a leading British medical journal, *The Lancet*, they examined forty controlled human studies of ginkgo and concluded that ginkgo was every bit as valid a treatment for "cerebral insufficiency" (decreased blood circulation in the brain that can lead to dementia) as the pharmaceutical drug co-dergocrine, widely prescribed in Europe for that condition. In fact, the Dutch researchers were so convinced of the efficacy of ginkgo that they vowed they would take it themselves if they ever began to lose their memory or experience other symptoms of "cerebral insufficiency." Moreover, they pronounced ginkgo free of serious side effects. The typical effective dose used in the studies: 120 milligrams daily. Improvements were generally noticeable after four to six weeks.

A NEW TREATMENT FOR ALZHEIMER'S

A common cause of age-related intellectual decline is the mysterious and dreaded disease Alzheimer's, in which brain cells are gradually destroyed. New, exciting research shows that ginkgo can help arrest the progression of dementia from Alzheimer's as well as from other causes. This does not mean the botanical drug cures the underlying cause of brain destruction or reverses brain damage, but several studies find much improvement in Alzheimer's patients taking ginkgo. In a large, very tightly structured study, published in 1996, German investigators at the Free University, Berlin, observed the use of ginkgo on 222 outpatients at forty-one study centers around the country. The subjects, all over age fifty-five, had been diagnosed with mild to moderate Alzheimer-type dementia or dementia caused by a series of mini strokes, known medically as multi-infarcts. For six months the patients were given either a dummy pill or a daily dose of 240 milligrams of standardized ginkgo biloba extract (EGb 761), taken twice a day before meals.

Undeniably, those getting ginkgo did much better. As judged by specific tests, overall condition, including improvement in "memory and attention functions," was about three times better in ginkgo takers than in those on the inactive pills. The plant medicine was more effective after six months than after three months. Moreover, side effects were infrequent and almost entirely minor, such as allergic reaction, upset stomach, or headache of the type related to any drug therapy; only one possible serious side effect occurred, a stroke, although the relationship to ginkgo was not confirmed. Using ginkgo to treat dementia could have monumental benefits for both the individual and society, the researchers concluded, by improving the patients' quality of life and postponing as long as possible the loss of independence and necessity for full-time care.

EXCITING NEW DISCOVERIES IN THE UNITED STATES

Dr. Turan M. Itil, a New York neuropsychiatrist, is a worldwide authority on the pharmacology of the brain. He is a leading pioneer in the development of pharmaceutical treatments for brain diseases. He chairs the World Health Organization's International Advisory Committee on the Diagnosis, Prevention, and Treatment of Alzheimer's Disease. Additionally, Dr. Itil is a clinical professor of psychiatry at New York University Medical Center and chairman of the New York Institute for Medical Research in Tarrytown. Dr. Itil takes ginkgo to protect his memory; so do his wife and "most of my friends over age sixty-five," he says. That's because the doctor is well acquainted with the power of ginkgo in the brain.

Dr. Itil has mapped the brain activity of ginkgo extract, has tested it on about 300 patients with significant memory disturbances, and is convinced it can stop or slow down the progression of memory loss, dementia, and Alzheimer's disease related to aging. "How can I in good conscience give ginkgo biloba to people if I don't believe in it enough to take it myself?" he asks. So persuasive is the evidence that Dr. Itil is calling for worldwide clinical trials of ginkgo to be partly funded by the U.S. government and carried out at about twenty of the World Health Organization's clinical centers around the world.

Dr. Itil knows ginkgo has striking pharmacological activity in the brain, as revealed by electroencephalograms (EEGs). In one test of the herb's effects on the central nervous system, he measured the brain wave activity of a group of healthy young males, average age thirty-two, after they had taken three brands of ginkgo. One brand, Ginkgold (a German product sold in the United States by Nature's Way), was active enough to be classified as a "cognitive activator," or "smart pill," on a par with prescription drugs. These cognitive activators are chemicals that can reverse disturbances in the memory and are used as psychotropic or "antidementia" pharmaceutical drugs. An hour after Ginkgold was ingested, alpha brain wave activity rose in all areas of the user's brain, the EEGs showed. Essentially the same thing happens after the subjects took tacrine, the first drug approved in the United States for treating dementia.

Next question: In a head-to-head test could ginkgo really work as well as pharmaceutical drugs to manipulate brain waves in the memory-impaired? Dr. Itil, again using EEGs, compared brain activity profiles in people given ginkgo and the drug tacrine. This time he used older men and women, average age sixty-seven, with memory problems, who had been diagnosed with mild to moderate dementia. The EEGs showed similar profiles of brain activity after the subjects took ginkgo or tacrine or several other "cognitive activating" antidementia drugs approved in Europe.

But ginkgo was superior; it decidedly led to brain changes in three times as many individuals. Alpha brain activity picked up, sometimes markedly, after three hours in 66 percent of the subjects taking a one-time dose of 240 milligrams of Ginkgold. That compared with only 22 percent of subjects taking tacrine. These tests lend much credibility to ginkgo's potential. Previous tests by Dr. Itil have shown that individuals in a confused, delirious state due to dementia have abnormal EEG readings that become normal after they take tacrine regularly; at the same time, their confusion and delirium disappear. Thus ginkgo's stronger ability to "normalize" EEG readings would predict that it might be even more effective than the approved risky prescription drug in reversing some aspects of fading mental abilities.

How Does It Work?
First, ginkgo is a very strong antioxidant, meaning it protects cells from damage, an underlying cause of all bodily disintegration, including dysfunctional brain cells and clogged blood vessels in the brain, heart, and extremities.

Ginkgo's main pharmacological agents are thought to be flavone glycosides and terpene lactones, mainly unique chemicals called ginkgolides. Ginkgo discourages blood platelet stickiness, reducing formation of devastating blood clots and plaque buildup. Also critical may be ginkgo's anti-inflammatory activity, which can protect diseased arteries from further damage, new research suggests. French experiments show that ginkgo can actually restore the ability of brain cells to transmit and receive signals from neurotransmitters that govern brain activity. Whether the direct therapeutic effects on the brain are ultimately the result of better blood circulation is unknown. Dr. Itil notes that ginkgo increases glucose (sugar) metabolism in the brain, thus increasing "brain energy. We don't know why this happens. It might be due to increased blood circulation in the brain, but I can't say for sure."

Remarkable new studies at the University of Kentucky by Dr. David Snowdon support that theory. In autopsies of the brains of elderly Catholic nuns diagnosed with Alzheimer's disease, Dr. Snowdon found that the cause of memory loss and dementia may not be entirely due to a peculiar damage to brain cells ("neuropathologic lesions") as previously thought, but to accompanying damage from infarcts or "mini strokes" in which blood flow is interrupted. This is exciting because it means the circulatory damage might be controlled even when the underlying disease of Alzheimer's is not. Thus the awful consequences of Alzheimer's may be treatable by preventing such "mini strokes," with aspirin and other anticoagulants and by improving blood circulation, as ginkgo does splendidly. Indeed, this helps confirm that increased blood flow to brain cells is the prime reason ginkgo is so successful in treating mental decline.

Who Should Take It?

Everybody who experiences memory disturbances might consider ginkgo as a way of trying to halt the gradual mental downslide into memory loss and possibly irreversible dementia. Waiting can be disastrous, says Dr. Itil. He points out that the longer you live, the more apt you are to experience a general decline in mental abilities, known medically by the frightening term "dementia." And those who develop memory problems earliest are most apt to be most severely impaired later. Individuals who develop memory problems in their forties and fifties, and particularly in their sixties and seventies, may decline into "probable" Alzheimer's disease five to ten years later. Overwhelmingly, most age-related dementia comes from vascular disease in the brain, including strokes, and the brain disease Alzheimer's. First signs are usually lapses in short-term memory, confusion, and personality changes, followed later by paranoia, depression, psychotic delusions, and possibly a return to a condition of infancy, requiring total care.

The time to start taking ginkgo is at the first signs of memory troubles, which are an indication that not all is right with the brain, according to Dr. Itil. Early intervention could dramatically forestall further brain deterioration.

What about ginkgo as a general brain protector after middle age? That may be a good idea, too, says Dr. Cott, age fifty, who takes ginkgo to help prevent memory decline. "I felt I was old enough to start," he says.

How Much Do You Need?

The well-tested effective dose for age-related loss of short-term memory and other mild signs of brain disturbances is a total of 120 milligrams daily, divided into three doses of 40-milligram pills. However, a higher dose is more effective, according to new research, on people with more serious dementia and Alzheimer's disease. The tested dose in such cases is a total of 240 milligrams daily. But it's not necessary to take the highest dose right away, say experts. It's better to start with a lower dose, look for improvement, and then work up to a higher dose if needed, says Dr. Itil.

How Quickly Does It Work?

Usually improvement in memory occurs in four to six weeks, although ginkgo has an instant effect on the brain: It revs up brain wave activity within an hour after it is taken, according to EEG studies on humans. Sometimes users become more coherent within an hour or so, according to reports.

However, ginkgo's benefits appear to accumulate over time and are greater at six months than at three months in cases of dementia, one large study found. "Be patient. The most dramatic changes may not appear for up to six months," says Dr. Itil. He also finds that ginkgo stays active in the brain for a long time. "We have seen up to nine hours' effect after a single dose of ginkgo," he reports.

The Safety Factor

Occasionally takers have complained of very mild and reversible side effects, such as upset stomach and headaches. One-half of 1 percent in a large study of 8,500 persons had such reactions. High doses of ginkgo may cause some dizziness at first. If dizziness occurs, experts recommend starting with a lower dose and building up to the higher dose.

Dr. Itil has never seen a serious side effect in about 300 patients he has treated with ginkgo; he considers it safer even than vitamin E, a vitamin with an excellent safety record. However, two new cases have been reported in the medical literature linking ginkgo with increased bleeding behind the eye and in the brain. Although the cause of these incidents has not been confirmed, ginkgo does prolong bleeding time and increase blood flow, and high doses might be contraindicated in those who are on anticoagulant medications or have uncontrolled high blood pressure, bleeding problems or a history of hemorrhagic stroke. In such cases medical supervision is advised when taking ginkgo.

Caution: If you have noticeable memory disturbances, consult a doctor immediately. It could be due to other causes, such as a brain tumor, that require medical treatment. Do not automatically assume you are suffering age-related memory decline that can be self-treated with ginkgo.

What's the Alternative?

Two antidementia prescription drugs are currently approved in this country, but are usually recommended as a last resort—only after memory loss and brain dysfunction are advanced, because of the drugs' severe side effects. There is no pharmaceutical equivalent of ginkgo that can be taken when you most need it—at the very earliest signs of memory disturbance or to prevent the age-related threat of memory loss.

> *How can you tell if ginkgo is working? The best measure is if you notice improvement in the memory or other day-to-day functioning of someone taking ginkgo. All the subtle pencil-and-paper tests and brain wave measurements are no substitute for that in the real world.*—Jerry Cott, Ph.D., National Institute of Mental Health

Consumer Concerns

Which type ginkgo is best? Not all ginkgo has the same potency. Of three brands tested by Dr. Itil, only Ginkgold had the potency of a pharmaceutical drug. All three samples bought in U.S. stores were properly standardized to contain 24 percent flavone glycosides and 6 percent terpenes.

Regardless, Ginkgold displayed greater bioavailability and pharmacological activity. Ginkgold is identical to EGb 761, a standardized ginkgo product, widely tested in Germany and France and approved by the German government for treating the symptoms of vascular and degenerative dementia, including memory deficits and disturbances in concentration, as well as tinnitus and intermittent claudication (leg pain from poor circulation). It is also sold in the United States under the brand name Ginkoba, from Pharmaton Natural Health Products.

What Else Is It Good For?

According to research, ginkgo appears to help ameliorate other neurological problems, such as head trauma, tinnitus of vascular origin, age-related depression, and certain cognitive symptoms of schizophrenia. Ginkgo has also been used to treat various cardiovascular problems, presumably by increasing blood flow; these include atherosclerosis, varicose veins, and intermittent claudication (pain in the calves of the legs from poor blood circulation).

The effects of increasing blood circulation with ginkgo can have far-reaching benefits. German urologists recently found ginkgo a good treatment for male impotence; the herbal treatment stimulated blood flow through penile arteries, promoting erections. Indeed, 78 percent of fifty men suffering from "arterial erectile impotence" improved after taking 240 milligrams of ginkgo biloba extract daily for nine months, researchers found. Blood flow to penile arteries generally improved after three months. Twenty men regained spontaneous erections after six months. Nineteen men regained potency when ginkgo was given with certain drug injections. Eleven remained impotent. In a previous study, the researchers had found some improvement from daily doses of only 60 milligrams of ginkgo. Neither dose caused any side effects.

Zaps Cholesterol, Unclogs Arteries

(GRAPEFRUIT FIBER)

It promises to lower your cholesterol more dramatically than anything else you can take, and it may clean out your arteries, too—all without the side effects of drugs.

It starts in childhood and progresses relentlessly until your arteries are wrecked—stiff, hard, and stuffed with plaque and debris. By middle age, most of us are hoping for a medical miracle to rescue us from the dreaded consequences of this premier killer, atherosclerosis. True, with a strict diet, drugs, exercise, and stress control, you may be able to stop the damage to your arteries from progressing. But what if you could swallow a magic powder to significantly reopen clogged arteries so blood can better flow through to the heart and brain, lessening your chances of heart attacks, bypass surgery, strokes, chest pain, and all the ills brought on by clogged arteries? And how about driving down cholesterol, when even the latest brainchild of the pharmaceutical industry has failed?

There is such a powder that more than one user has dubbed a miracle.

S. L. GARRETT'S MIRACLE
"How My Arteries Unclogged Without Drugs or Surgery"

At age seventy S. L. Garrett had little reason to worry about a stroke or heart attack. His blood cholesterol was normal. An exam, several years earlier, triggered by slight chest pain, had uncovered no heart problems. Then in December 1994 he had an alarming disturbance of vision in his left eye, signaling a TIA, or transient ischemic attack, a common prelude to stroke. Doctors first did a CT scan, finding no brain damage, and then ordered an ultrasound of his carotid arteries, leading up the sides of the neck to the brain. They suspected a blockage. Sure enough, resonating in the left artery was that characteristic sound, or bruit, a distinctive whoosh, indicating restricted blood flow. An arteriogram, in which a catheter is inserted at the base of the neck to take X-ray pictures of the carotid arteries, confirmed that Garrett's left carotid artery was 40 percent closed with plaque. And there were signs of ulceration, damage to the artery's interior walls. His right carotid artery was clogged to a lesser extent. The narrowing was not enough to warrant balloon surgery (an endocardectomy) to open it, but it was worrisome. If the artery clogging progressed, the next event could be a full-blown stroke. The recommended therapy: Take anticoagulants to increase blood flow, and medically monitor the condition.

Garrett, fearing the side effects of the anticoagulant, didn't like the idea. And aspirin, another blood-thinning possibility, was out of the question because he is allergic to it.

His son, S. W. "Wayne" Garrett, M.D., a radiologist at Columbia Putnam Medical Center in Patatka, Florida, suggested an alternative. He knew of experiments with grapefruit pectin, a fiber, conducted by Dr. James Cerda at the University of Florida, showing that pectin might clear out arteries. In fact, Cerda had been his professor in medical school. Dr. Garrett also knew the fiber dramatically lowered cholesterol. "Just to show Dad it was okay, I decided to try the pectin myself for a month—and I had a life insurance exam coming up, so I figured, how can it hurt?" said Dr. Garrett. He also liked the fact that unlike other cholesterol-reducing or cardiac drugs, the fiber has no dangerous side effects.

So he took Dr. Cerda's grapefruit fiber for a month and was stunned by the result. "My cholesterol, which ordinarily runs 180 to 200, dived to 150. More important, my HDLs [good cholesterol] jumped so high, they surpassed my LDLs [bad cholesterol]. My ratio was incredible—under one. I was amazed, really amazed it was that good." (The lower the ratio of LDLs or total cholesterol to HDLs, the lower the risk of heart disease. A ratio of under one is highly unusual and protective, especially in men.)

The senior Garrett, impressed, started taking the grapefruit fiber in January 1995—three times a day, usually mixed into water or juice. Sixteen months later, in May 1996, he underwent another ultrasound examination of his carotid arteries. Their interior landscape had changed dramatically. The plaque had shrunk, actually regressed more than one-third—down from a 40 percent closure to a 25 percent closure in the left carotid artery. The arterial walls, once bumpy with the plaque's debris, were much smoother and flatter. The ulceration was almost gone. Because the opening of the arteries had expanded so much, the blood flow through the arteries was "excellent."

Where did the plaque go? Obviously it was somehow dislodged, dissolved, swept away by the action of the grapefruit fiber. "No question, since Dad did nothing else different, it has to be the fiber," says his son the physician. Further, the grapefruit fiber surely helped clear other arteries in the body, because it does not target one specific blood vessel. "I feel more energetic than I've felt in years," says S.L. Garrett.

Is it a miracle? It certainly seems like one to many who use it. Nobody can think of a pharmaceutical drug that could have caused the entrenched plaque to disappear, opening the arteries. The most such drugs do, if you're lucky, is to preserve the status quo so arteries don't get worse. But actually reverse the clogging? Medical consensus says it's unlikely, if not impossible, especially in such a short time and especially with something as benign as grapefruit fiber. Dr. Cerda agrees that "if a new pharmaceutical drug did the same thing—removed one-third of the plaque from old beaten-up arteries, the makers would declare it a miracle cure, sell it for a trillion dollars, and everybody would want it."

JOAN'S MIRACLE
A 90-Point Cholesterol Dive in One Month

Joan Levin has a master's degree in public health from Johns Hopkins University as well as a law degree, so when her cholesterol began to climb steadily after age fifty, she knew what to do: She went on every cholesterol-controlling regimen she could find. "I tried everything—very rigorous low-fat diets and exercise, but nothing made a dent. I was afraid to take drugs like Mevacor and Zocor because of side effects—liver damage. Anything that affects liver metabolism, as these drugs do, scared me." Still, her cholesterol was going up, up, up, and her physician insisted that cholesterol-lowering drugs were her only option because nothing else worked.

In the summer of 1996 she heard about a special grapefruit fiber product. She started taking it dissolved in water. Although the directions said to take it three times a day, she took it usually twice a day, always being careful to get the full day's recommended dose. After a month she had her blood cholesterol tested. When she got the report in the mail it was so unbelievable, she actually let out a yelp. Her cholesterol had dived from 295 to 208! "The LDL [bad cholesterol] and the triglycerides went down about 100 points. It was just fantastic, really miraculous. I can't see why anyone would want to start hazardous cholesterol drugs before trying this. If it doesn't work after a month, you know it, and can then go on to something else."

And the grapefruit fiber had some fabulous unexpected side effects: After three months on grapefruit fiber, Joan had, without trying, trimmed 15 pounds off her five-foot-eight-inch, 160-pound body. "I realized after a couple of weeks of taking the fiber I wasn't that hungry anymore. I was losing weight very gradually. And I don't have these mad, mad food cravings anymore." Moreover, her energy level has skyrocketed. Never known as a jock, Joan has taken up fast-walking, and in the fall won a medal for second place in her age group among 350 contestants in a Chicago race. I beat all the men in my age group. This stuff has changed my life."

Joan continues to take the grapefruit fiber, hoping to get her cholesterol down to 180. Many people she tells about it are enthusiastic, including some of her medical and scientific friends. But others whom it might help, she laments, are skeptical. "Unfortunately, we've been so totally brainwashed that most people think the only thing that can help us is a patented product prescribed by a physician," she says. "Everything else is immediately suspect. It's really too bad, because I think this could help a lot of people."

A HEART SURGEON'S
MOTHER'S MIRACLE
"I Gave Up Mevacor for Grapefruit Fiber"

Dr. Daniel Knauf, a vascular surgeon on the faculty of the University of Florida College of Medicine, says that his seventy-six-year-old mother's cholesterol dropped to its lowest point in recent years, below 200, after she took grapefruit fiber. Thus she was able to totally quit her cholesterol-lowering drugs;

she had been on cholesterol-lowering Provochal for five years and Mevacor for six months, and these were not as effective as the grapefruit fiber. Further, Mevacor produced signs of liver damage. She has happily kept her cholesterol down for two years with grapefruit fiber alone, prompting her heart surgeon son to joke that this stuff "could put me out of business."

What Is It?

The special grapefruit fiber mixture that opened Garrett's arteries and lowered Joan Levin's cholesterol is a unique form of pectin—a water-soluble fiber, obtained mostly from the rinds, membranes, and juice sacs of the grapefruit, and combined with another soluble fiber, guar gum. It is processed into a pale yellow, tasteless powder to be dissolved in liquids or sprinkled on food. It is patented by the University of Florida and by Dr. James Cerda and is commercially called ProFibe.

What's the Evidence?

Literally dozens of excellent studies in the United States and elsewhere have found that soluble fiber and its by-products in various foods, including beta glucans in oats and pectin in fruit, can all lower blood cholesterol. Following that lead, Dr. James J. Cerda, a gastroenterologist and professor of medicine at the University of Florida College of Medicine, for twenty years has focused on the unique powers of pectin, a soluble fiber in grapefruit, to save and restore arteries. Dr. Cerda's first breakthrough experiment in 1988 showed that grapefruit pectin dramatically lowered cholesterol in miniature pigs put on a high-fat diet. The pig's cardiovascular system is almost identical to that of a human. Cerda fed the pigs a diet with 15 per-cent lard (equal to about 40 percent of calories in fat). Predictably their cholesterol soared and their arteries closed. But when the pigs also ate pectin, their blood cho-lesterol fell 20 to 25 percent. Still, that was not the biggest surprise. When Dr. Cerda examined their arteries under the microscope, he was incredulous. The arteries of the pectin-fed pigs were much less clogged and generally much healthier.

Dr. Cerda suspected that grapefruit pectin, regardless of lowering cholesterol, could also prevent and even reverse artery clogging. So for another year fifteen new pigs were fed lots of lard. Then Dr. Cerda added grapefruit fiber to half the pigs' fatty diets. Nine months later the pigs were sacrificed and their arteries and hearts painstak-ingly examined. "It was so exciting," exclaims Dr. Cerda. The arteries of the pigs fed pectin were much healthier, revealing little of the destruction to arteries—the hunks of plaque stuck in artery walls and narrowed arteries able to accommodate only trickles of blood—found in pigs not fed pectin. The researchers measured the amount of arter-ial surface area covered by plaque and diameters of arter-ial openings. The astonishing finding: The pectin-fed pigs had fully 60 percent less atherosclerosis in their coronary arteries and aortas. That meant pectin was a remarkable healer of arteries, opening and smoothing them out, or a strong block to the progression of atherosclerosis. Or both.

EVERYBODY'S CHOLESTEROL FALLS

In humans, Dr. Cerda has documented that grapefruit fiber reduces cholesterol in virtually everyone to some degree. In one study he measured the cholesterol of the first 100 patients who consecutively came to the heart clinic at the hospital where he practices. He encouraged all of them to start on 15 grams (about a third of a cup) of grapefruit fiber daily. "What we found was incredible," says Dr. Cerda. "Their cholesterol, usually in the range of 220 to 300, dropped very quickly as much as 25 to 30 percent in one month!" In some people with exceptionally high cholesterol, grapefruit fiber does reduce it, but not enough to make doctors happy. In such cases a combination of standard cholesterol-lowering drugs, such as Mevacor and Zocor, plus grapefruit fiber may work. A small unpublished study of seven patients with cholesterol of 350 to 400 found that either grapefruit pectin alone or drugs alone brought it down to 225 to 300. On standard doses of both the grapefruit pectin and drugs, the cholesterol frequently dropped below 200.

Human tests of grapefruit fiber's ability to open up arteries, reversing atherosclerosis, are soon to get under way on 200 patients with diseased carotid arteries at several centers around the United States. In a double-blind test, half will get real grapefruit fiber (ProFibe) and half will get a look-alike inactive powder (placebo) for eighteen to twenty-four months. Any regression or clearing of the arteries will be detected by ultrasound.

How Does It Work?
The exact mechanisms by which soluble fiber reduces cholesterol are not clear. Some theories: The fiber creates an ultra-thin layer of water in the intestinal tract, hindering absorption of cholesterol-raising fat; the fiber produces by-product chemicals that suppress the liver's production of cholesterol, somewhat the way prescription drugs do. How grapefruit fiber might dissolve plaque buildup and open up arteries is more mysterious. Dr. Cerda speculates that a unique polysaccharide, galactur-

onic acid, in grapefruit chemically interacts with the destructive stuff in arteries, including bad LDL cholesterol, to prevent and break up plaque deposits.

There's also some evidence that aggressive lowering of cholesterol, as shown with drugs, tends to open arteries, improve blood flow, and cause a regression of atherosclerosis. But Cerda is convinced that grapefruit fiber's ability to diminish plaque in arteries is independent of its cholesterol-lowering capabilities.

How Much Do You Need?

The standard dose used in clinical studies is about one-third of a cup a day, or 15 grams of fiber, divided into three doses taken at breakfast, lunch, and dinner. This much may be needed to achieve a regression of plaque in arteries. However, many people get a dramatic cholesterol drop from just 5 grams (one scoop) or 10 grams (two scoops) daily, says Dr. Cerda.

The Safety Factor

Many users have gas, especially until they adapt to the high-fiber intake. Also, loose stools are common and, in some cases, diarrhea. You can reduce the dose or start on a lower dose and work up to a larger dose as your body adapts to the high fiber. Because it is a fruit fiber, there is no long-term toxicity.

What's the Alternative?

Popular cholesterol-reducing drugs, such as Mevacor and Zocor, are effective in many people, but are more costly than grapefruit fiber and can have serious side effects, including liver damage; regular liver function tests are needed to detect damage when such drugs are taken. California cardiologist Dean Ornish has reported some regression of atherosclerosis with a stringent low-fat diet, exercise, and stress reduction. Garlic can also help lower cholesterol, and antioxidants may help prevent plaque deposits and partially restore arteries to health. Otherwise, the only way to open severely clogged arteries is by surgery.

Consumer Concerns
ProFibe grapefruit powder is available in some health food stores, drugstores, and supermarkets. For mail orders, call 800–756–3999. It costs about $60 a month for the maximum dose, or $2 a day. A small scoop to measure doses is included with each container.

Should You Try It?
If you are worried about the state of your cholesterol and arteries, it is surely worth a try. It seems to be almost an instant supercure for high cholesterol in many people, forcing cholesterol down 50 points or more after a month or two. The fiber also may help shrink the amount of plaque in arteries. Always consult with your doctor about the proper course of action. Self-medicating for heart disease without professional advice can be dangerous.

Note: You cannot get the same benefit from eating lots of grapefruit.

Nature's Mighty Aspirin

(FEVERFEW)

Why continue to suffer with migraines when a common herb can make them disappear?

As any sufferer of migraine knows, aspirin is a wimp against this ferocious headache. But nature has another secret potion that stops such headaches. Its users call it a "miracle aspirin"—a 10-cent pill with the awesome power to shut out those indescribably painful and incapacitating thunderstorms of the brain that afflict 23 million Americans. The cure is in the leaves of a plant called feverfew. And undeniably it works, as affirmed by thousands of migraine sufferers who have been lucky enough to try it.

THERESA'S MIRACLE
"Twenty Years of Pain and Misery—Gone!"

For more than twenty years, Theresa Colonna, now sixty-one and living in a suburb of Pittsburgh, was a prisoner of migraine headaches. They struck about once a week, usually spoiling weekends and holidays with her husband and four kids. "The migraines were so awful, everybody dreaded them. I usually had to go to bed for a day or two," she says. She suffered all the classic symptoms—visual disturbances, light sensitivity, slurred speech, throbbing head pain, and nausea. "Sometimes I just sat in the bathroom all day, throwing up."

To relieve her distress, she tried every offering of orthodox medicine. When the headaches were extra bad, she went to the emergency room. "They would give me a shot of Demerol and send me home to sleep it off." One doctor put her on Inderal, a beta blocker used to treat high blood pressure and often prescribed to prevent migraines. It didn't help. "I went to a chiropractor. I tried every drug on the market." In real emergencies she used a new injectible drug, sumatriptan (Imitrex), to stop the headache. When she felt a migraine coming on, she raced to her doctor for a quick-acting shot. "One time I went to his office wearing sunglasses to keep the light out and I could barely walk, but I had to attend a wedding. The shot was a godsend," she says. But that was her last severe migraine and an end to her need for conventional medicines. She discovered the herbal remedy feverfew.

Her boss, the principal of the school where she works as a secretary, sent her a magazine clipping about the herb. Skeptical but willing to try anything, she bought some feverfew tablets at her mall's health food store—Nature's Herbs, 100 capsules of 380 milligrams each for $10. "I took one pill three times a day for three months," she says. "It only cost 10 cents a pill. Now I take only one a day. It was just amazing. I had tried everything possible, and this little pill took my migraines away. Now I may get a headache every six months instead of once a week, but they're nothing like they were—not very severe and they don't last long. Actually I haven't had one for an entire year!"

She's aware of new Imitrex prescription pills that can knock out migraines once they start—and she even keeps some in a drawer, just in case a bad one strikes. "But I'm afraid of the side effects and I'd rather not take a drug every week to stop a headache when I can prevent it so easily without any side effects. And it's so much cheaper than the drugs. I feel so good, I'm afraid not to take feverfew," she says.

Recently Theresa went to a local meeting where a neurologist presented slides on all the drugs available to treat migraines. At the end she asked him if he had ever heard of feverfew. He said, "No. What is it?" "I tried to tell him, but he didn't seem interested," says Theresa. "He brushed it off as nothing important, even though several people in the audience said they were using it, too. I guess he only cared about prescribing strong drugs, which is too bad."

What Is It?

An ancient remedy, feverfew is a common feathery plant, a member of the daisy family. Since early Greek times it's been used to treat the same disorders as aspirin— headaches, fever, and rheumatic inflammations. In the 1600s British doctors proclaimed it "very effectual for all paines [sic] in the head." Physician John Hill in his book *The Family Herbal* in 1772 declared, "In the worst headache this herb exceeds whatever else is known." But feverfew fell into disuse for a few centuries—for one reason, despite its name, it wasn't very effective against fevers. It regained respectability in the 1980s when British researchers discovered it really is potent medicine against migraines.

What's the Evidence?

Some of the credit for making feverfew medically respectable goes to a British woman, a Mrs. Jenkins, who in the late 1970s cured her own migraines and triggered the first modern scientific validation of feverfew. She was the wife of the chief medical officer of Britain's National Coal Board. Age sixty-eight at the time, she had suffered migraine headaches for more than fifty years, since age sixteen. As the story goes, an acquaintance suggested she try an old folk remedy—chewing feverfew leaves—to cure her headaches. She started consuming three leaves a day, a dose rumored to work. Indeed it did. Her headaches became less frequent and less severe, and after ten months they were gone.

Her doctor husband passed the news along to Dr. E. Stewart Johnson at the City of London Migraine Clinic, who was intrigued and decided to look into the use of this popular migraine folk medicine. He located nearly 300 migraine sufferers who were regular users of feverfew leaves and questioned them. Their stories were so convincing that he and other researchers were prompted to conduct studies, published in Britain's top medical journals, showing that feverfew can help cure migraines.

In 1985 Dr. Johnson reported the results of his investigations in the prestigious *British Medical Journal*. In his survey of 270 migraine sufferers, 72 percent who chewed feverfew leaves claimed to have fewer and milder migraines. Dr. Johnson then decided to find out if their beliefs had any physical basis or were purely imaginary. He took seventeen migraine sufferers who regularly ate feverfew leaves to keep migraines away. He made test capsules with dried powdered feverfew and look-alike dummy capsules with no feverfew. The subjects, without knowing which they were taking, were assigned to take either a fake or a real capsule every day for about six months and record their migraine experience. The results were striking and convincing, showing that the activity of feverfew was real. Those actually getting the feverfew were relatively migraine-free, as before. But those suddenly deprived of feverfew were in agony. Their headaches tripled and were so incapacitating that some quit the study. When they resumed feverfew, their migraines diminished or vanished.

The clincher evidence for feverfew came from another so-called double-blind controlled study of migraine sufferers who had never before used feverfew. It was reported in the British medical journal *The Lancet* in 1988 by researchers from University Hospital in Nottingham, England. For two periods of four months, migraine sufferers took either a daily capsule of air-dried feverfew leaves (about two medium-sized leaves) or dried cabbage leaves, as a placebo or dummy pill. Again, the feverfew was a remarkable success; when subjects were taking the real herb, migraine occurrence dropped by one-fourth and headaches were much milder, with less vomiting and visual disturbance. That's why today you can find processed feverfew compressed into tablets and packed into capsules that equal pharmaceutical prescription drugs as antidotes to the curse of migraine headaches.

I have virtually wiped out the need to treat migraines in my patient population by telling them to try fever-

few.—Daniel Tucker, M.D., board-certified internist, immunologist, and allergist, West Palm Beach, Florida

How Does It Work?

Feverfew's most likely antimigraine agent is parthenolide. And many experts say feverfew must have relatively high concentrations of this chemical to be effective. Parthenolide has been shown to block the release of serotonin. An excess of serotonin, a hormone active in cells and blood vessels of the brain, is implicated in triggering migraines, most likely by constricting blood vessels. Thus feverfew appears to work much like the drug Sansert (methysergide maleate), a serotonin antagonist, designed to prevent migraines.

Feverfew, tests show, also has an anti-inflammatory effect that may be related to triggering migraines. Recent British research finds that feverfew's complex mix of chemicals are "high potency" inhibitors of thromboxane B2 and leukotriene B4, bodily substances that foster inflammation and pain. Indeed, feverfew leaves block the release of such inflammatory chemicals by 58 percent in test tube studies, explaining feverfew's anti-inflammatory effect. It also has antithrombotic activity, antibacterial activity, and antiallergic activity (it inhibits mast cell release of histamine.)

How Much Do You Need?

If you eat the dried leaves, two or three a day are considered an effective dose. Feverfew capsules or tablets usually contain at least 300 milligrams of the herb. The label recommends three a day. This is okay to start with, but one a day is often enough, say experts, to prevent onset of migraines.

The Safety Factor

Generally side effects of feverfew are few and very mild—minor mouth sores and gastrointestinal upset in about 8 percent of users, according to one study. Rare allergic reactions and rapid heartbeat in a few users have also been reported. Because of its centuries-long use the herb is considered nontoxic in the short term, but no long-term scientific studies have been done on its chronic use. In Canada, where feverfew is approved as a nonprescription drug for migraines, health authorities recommend that regular use as a prophylactic—more than four months at a time—be supervised by a physician. Dr. Michael Murray, Seattle naturopathic doctor, advises against using feverfew together with nonsteroidal anti-inflammatory drugs (NSAIDS), including aspirin and Tylenol, saying that they can reduce the herb's effectiveness.

Who Should Not Take It?

Pregnant women, (because it might cause uterine contractions), lactating mothers, and children under age two should not take feverfew. Be cautious if you are on anticoagulants, because feverfew has blood-thinning properties and could interact to promote bleeding in rare cases. Feverfew may trigger allergies in those who are also sensitive to ragweed.

Consumer Concerns

Since the leaves are bitter, a capsule or tablet is more agreeable and reliable than feverfew leaves. To be effective, pills should be "standardized" to contain the proper amount of the pharmacological agent, parthenolide. A high-quality feverfew preparation should contain 0.2 percent parthenolide (250 micrograms,), says herbal authority Dr. Varro Tyler. In one reported analysis, two out of three feverfew products bought in a Louisiana health food store had no parthenolide at all. Keep feverfew in the refrigerator to prevent its deterioration.

Should You Try It?

If you have migraines, feverfew should be your first "remedy of choice," because it can block headaches from occurring and reduce their severity with far less risk of side effects than prescription pharmaceuticals, and it is much less expensive. If it works, it's a miracle for you, too. If it doesn't, you can try other alternatives, including orthodox drugs, with nothing lost and no harm done.

What Else Is It Good For?

The British widely use feverfew to reduce the pain of rheumatoid arthritis. It makes sense pharmacologically; rheumatoid arthritis symptoms flare up when cells are flooded with leukotrienes, inflammatory agents curbed by feverfew constituents. No good clinical studies back up feverfew's efficacy for arthritis, and thus an effective dose is unclear. (One study found no effect, but the dose may have been too low.) Feverfew has also been touted to relieve asthma, allergies, dermatitis, and psoriasis. All are characterized by inflammatory reactions, providing some rationale for the treatment. How well feverfew works for such conditions is unknown, because of the lack of clinical tests.

Wonder Drug
for Osteoarthritis

(GLUCOSAMINE)

It's the only agent known that can stop or reverse the biggest crippler of all—osteoarthritis. And it's totally safe!

No wonder arthritis sufferers call it a "wonder drug." It decidedly is when pitted against the alternatives offered by conventional medicine—"gnarled joints, inexorable pain, and little hope for a cure," as one expert aptly put it. A natural substance called glucosamine, sometimes combined with another nutrient, chondroitin, is the most potent medicine, prescription or other, known to combat the underlying cause of joint degeneration, most often exemplified by osteoarthritis, the crippler that strikes nearly 90 percent of us if we live long enough.

Here's what happens: The articular cartilage—that smooth, tough, rubbery, gelatinous stuff that acts as a cushion or shock absorber to keep the ends of the bones in your joints from rubbing together—begins to break down and doesn't regenerate. (It's like the cartilage mass you see on the end of a chicken drumstick.) It deteriorates and dries out like an old ragged piece of foam that has lost its bounce; attacked by enzymes, cartilage disintegrates, cracking and even disappearing in serious cases, leaving the ends of bones uncovered. As cartilage disappears, pain appears, joints stiffen, and mobility lessens. It is a dismal condition that progresses, attacking one joint after another, mainly in the fingers, knees, and hips, with no apparent cure.

The commonly prescribed treatment: painkillers such as acetaminophen (Tylenol), aspirin, and stronger nonsteroidal antiinflammatory drugs or NSAIDS, such as indomethacin (Indocin) and ibuprofen (Motrin, Advil, Aleve), that can cause ulcers, gastrointestinal bleeding, and kidney damage if you use them long enough. Even worse, few people realize that these recommended painkillers actually tend to destroy cartilage and discourage the production of new cartilage, according to recent Italian evidence. The common palliative, then, not only does not address the underlying cause of osteoarthritis but actually makes it worse, although with the pain diminished, most people are not aware of the real nature of what's happening to them.

But what if you could build cartilage back up, actually regenerate it? Conventional American medicine says osteoarthritis cannot be reversed, and in most cases not even arrested—only treated with powerful analgesics and anti-inflammatories to mask the pain and, as a last resort, with surgical joint replacement. Yet that's not the medical consensus in other countries. In Europe patients with osteoarthritis are routinely given special nutrients—glucosamine and chondroitins—to stimulate the growth of new cartilage, stemming the progression of osteoarthritis and even reversing it. Some American doctors and patients are now using these nutrients with incredible success. Still, millions of Americans are being deprived of a sensible, safe, relatively inexpensive hope for recovery because they don't know it exists.

PHYLLIS'S MIRACLE
"I Escaped Hip Replacement Surgery"

Not yet fifty years old in 1989, Phyllis Eagelton,* a high-powered Washington attorney with a private firm, found herself in severe pain; the joints and muscles of her left hip were disintegrating. She hobbled so badly that she had to use a cane. "I couldn't walk more than a block or two without pain," she recalls. Overseas trips to engage in international negotiations were extremely difficult. Tennis, which she loved and had played since she was a child, became unthinkable. She consulted medical experts. X-rays confirmed a severe loss of cartilage and bone abnormalities in the joint of her left hip. The diagnosis: osteoarthritis that was progressive and untreatable except for painkillers and surgery. Reluctantly she went on powerful nonsteroidial anti-inflammatory drugs called NSAIDS, at the recommendation of a rheumatologist. She felt "somewhat better" but quit after a few weeks, fearing side effects. Two orthopedic surgeons in Washington, D.C., recommended hip replacement surgery, warning that otherwise her disability would progress to the point where she could not walk.

She rejected it. "My view was if I had severe arthritis in my hip, it would appear elsewhere and that replacing one joint was not a total solution." She began searching for alternatives, trying chiropractic manipulations, various Chinese herbs, black currant oil, acupuncture, and stretching and exercise to lessen the pain and increase mobility. They all seemed to help somewhat, but, fortunately, she also learned about a natural antiarthritic substance called glucosamine, recommended by Stanford-trained Washington physician Robert Heffron. She started taking the pill and noticed a lessening of pain within three weeks, followed by remarkable improvement over the next few months. "It really kicked in for her," says Dr. Heffron, who has recommended it for many patients, including his brother, a professional baseball player with osteoarthritis of the knee.

Phyllis has now been using a combination of glucosamine, chondroitin-sulfates, and manganese (Cosamin) for two years with what she calls miraculous results. Her crippling arthritis has diminished to the point that she barely notices it. She walks without difficulty. She does not take aspirin or other analgesics. The cane is gone, and so is the pain. "I still don't have all the flexibility I want, but I'm essentially pain-free," she says. "Last summer I played tennis for the first time in eight years— something I thought I would never do again—and kept it up three times a week. It was wonderful. I also went hiking last year in Arizona; I walked five or six miles at a stretch without pain. I would say I can walk on a flat hard surface indefinitely."

Obviously a hip replacement operation is now far from Phyllis's mind. "It's out of the question," says Dr. Heffron. But her insurance company has still not forgiven her. Although she is no longer disabled at all by arthritis, the company will not renew her health insurance because she refused to have the recommended hip replacement surgery—which, of course, she doesn't need now, since she defied conventional opinion by recovering without it.

*A pseudonym has been used to protect privacy, but the medical details are accurate.

What Is It?

Glucosamine (glue-KOSE-ah-mean) is a nutrient found in very small amounts in food; it is also made by the cartilage cells of the body. Its main job is to prod the production of long chains of sugars called glycosaminoglycans (GAGs), necessary to rebuild cartilage. Since 1992 veterinarians have been using synthetic glucosamine as a dietary supplement to treat arthritis in racehorses, farm animals, and pets. Some arthritis sufferers and doctors have been inspired to try glucosamine after it worked in their dogs. Chondroitin (con-DROY-tin) is another major cartilage builder and is made into supplements from cow, shark, and whale cartilage.

What's the Evidence?

Glucosamine has been the "drug of choice" for treating osteoarthritis in Portugal, Spain, and Italy since the early 1980s. No question, when swallowed, the substances rapidly reach the proper targets—connective tissues and joint cartilage, as tracked by the use of radioactively labeled agents. Five rigorously conducted double-blind studies done in the 1980s on glucosamine alone show impressive results. One study by Italian investigators at Giustinian Hospital in Venice found that glucosamine reduced overall symptoms of chronic osteoarthritis by 80 percent after only twenty-one days; improvement was noticeable in seven days. One quarter of the patients became symptom-free after three weeks of treatment.

In another high-quality controlled study of patients with osteoarthritis of the knee, done at the National

Orthopedic Hospital in Manila, Philippines, 80 to 100 percent of those given glucosamine improved, usually within two weeks. Particularly remarkable and convincing is a study at the University of Pavia and Rota Research Laboratories in Italy, in which eighty patients hospitalized with flare-ups of osteoarthritis (of the neck, lumbar spine, or multiple joints) took either 1,500 milligrams daily of glucosamine sulfate or a dummy pill (placebo.) Physicians rated glucosamine about twice as effective as the placebo, with 72 percent of glucosamine takers judged "excellent or good" after three weeks. About 20 percent were free of pain and other symptoms.

Most revealing, researchers took samples of hip and knee cartilage from patients on glucosamine or placebo and examined them under an electron microscope. The difference was startling. The cartilage of placebo takers displayed the typical cavities and rough fibrous surfaces characteristic of severe osteoarthritis. In contrast, the cartilage of glucosamine-treated patients "showed almost smooth cartilage surfaces," and only minor signs of osteoarthritis. The study provides direct visual evidence that glucosamine actually repaired cartilage, in other words attacked the underlying cause of the osteoarthritis; further, the cartilage regeneration happened within thirty days!

BETTER THAN MOTRIN

Moreover, research in Portugal, Germany, and Italy has found that, for relieving symptoms, glucosamine is equal to or better than typical drugs prescribed in the United States, mainly ibuprofen (known as Advil, Motrin, or Nuprin). In a Portuguese study of forty patients, Dr. Antonio Lopes Vaz, at Oporto's St. John Hospital, found that ibuprofen produced faster pain relief in the first two weeks. But after eight weeks the glucosamine group had on average a threefold lower pain score than the ibuprofen takers. In 20 percent taking glucosamine, swelling of the knee disappeared, compared with no loss of swelling in the ibuprofen group. Overall the glucosamines worked better than ibuprofen to relieve pain and swelling in 29 percent of the patients.

In a large nine-month study at several medical centers in Portugal 252 doctors compared glucosamine sulfate (1,500 milligrams daily) with other common treatments in 1,506 osteoarthritis patients. Glucosamine beat out anti-inflammatory agents, injectible cartilage extracts, vitamins, and all other oral agents, bringing improvement in 95 percent of subjects, even in many who had not responded to any other medical treatment. Only 5 percent did not improve. The researchers concluded that "oral treatment with glucosamine sulfate manages most arthrosis [arthritic] patients to full or partial recovery."

Glucosamine also proved more effective than piroxicam, a popular European arthritis drug, in a 1994 study. Dr. Luigi Rovati at the Rotta Research Laboratories in Italy, who discovered the glucosamine sulfate molecule in the early 1960s, found glucosamine more effective in dampening disease activity in 329 patients with osteoarthritis than either a placebo or piroxicam alone or in combination with glucosamine.

What also makes glucosamine vastly superior is the lack of side effects. For example, in Dr. Rovati's latest study, 15 percent of the patients on glucosamine complained of side effects compared with 41 percent on the drug piroxicam and 24 percent on placebo. Another 1994 study of 200 patients in three German centers and one Italian center found that glucosamine sulfate suppressed pain as well as ibuprofen did. However, 35 percent taking ibuprofen complained of adverse effects, compared with 6 percent taking glucosamines.

EXCITING NEW PROOF IN THE UNITED STATES

Dr. Amal Das, an orthopedic surgeon specializing in knee and hip replacements in Hendersonville, North Carolina, was excited over an article a few years ago in a European medical journal, reporting successes in thousands of patients from a new agent that slowed down the progression of osteoarthritis. "I was thrilled, because I've been looking for biological alternatives to joint replacement. The medications we use in the U.S. don't really slow down the progression of arthritis; all they do is treat the pain." Dr. Das was particularly intrigued by a European study showing that the natural agents reduced the need for joint replacement by two-thirds in a group of patients.

Dr. Das did a computer search of the U.S. medical literature and could not find a single study on the use of the agents glucosamine or chondroitin in treating arthritis. He determined to do a study of his own, using the highest scientific standards. Two years ago, on the basis of the European evidence, he started a pilot study using the agents on some of his osteoarthritic patients, particularly those who had serious side effects from anti-inflammatory drugs.

Although he stresses that the evidence is anecdotal, it was extremely impressive. Many of his patients, like those in the European studies, improved dramatically. "I've had several patients whose pain has been alleviated." He has also put off replacing the joints of several patients because the glucosamine-chondroitin combination made the surgery unnecessary. "We have a physical therapist in the hospital who had severe pain in both knees; it's now gone." Dr. Das's own father, also a physician, who suffers with severe osteoarthritis in his knees, has eased his pain by taking the agents.

But the real proof? Does Dr. Das see X-ray evidence

that the glucosamine-chrondroitin has actually stimulated the growth of new cartilage, in effect reversing osteo-arthritis? "Yes. I have seen radiographic evidence of improvement." Previously Dr. Das was skeptical of European claims of cartilage regeneration. He explains that severe osteoarthritis is characterized on X-ray by a narrowing of the joint space as cartilage disappears and bones come closer together. "Some European studies show that joint space has regenerated, but I have tended never to believe it. Now I must admit I have seen a normalization of the joint spaces on the X-rays of some of my patients who have been on the medication for a year." This is irrefutable evidence that new cartilage has appeared, in a sense healing the damage and reversing the disease.

All this has caused Dr. Das to begin the first U.S. double-blind placebo-controlled study of 100 patients with mild to severe osteoarthritis of the knees or hips, using a glucosamine-chondroitin sulfate combination, Cosamin DS. "Since at least eighteen European studies already show [glucosamine's] effectiveness, we're not discovering anything; we're just stealing from Europe," says Dr. Das. "But it's just that U.S. physicians don't believe European studies until they're repeated here." Dr. Das's study should be completed in 1998.

How Does It Work?
Glucosamine works mainly by stimulating the rebuilding of damaged cartilage. It also affects metabolism of cartilage in ways to prevent its breakdown. Additionally, it has some anti-inflammatory activity, but basically it relieves pain, swelling, and tenderness by rebuilding stiff and eroded joint tissue, which is the cause of the pain in the first place. Chondroitin actually draws fluid into cartilage, important because the fluid attracts nutrients and helps hydrate the

cartilage, making it more spongy. Chondroitins protect old cartilage from premature degeneration and act as building blocks for the creation of healthy new cartilage.

In extensive European research, glucosamine alone, mainly in the form of glucosamine sulfate, has been found extremely effective, but some experts believe that the addition of chondroitins makes even more powerful medicine.

How Much Do You Need?
To make it easy, you can simply follow the doses recommended on the label. These are generally adequate for most people. If you want to be more precicse, you can follow the guidelines of Jason Theodosakis, M.D., who has used the agents on himself and about 600 patients, as noted in his bestselling book *The Arthritis Cure* (St. Martin's Press, 1997). Here are doses he advises, based on your body weight: "Less than 120 pounds: 1,000 milligrams of glucosamine and 800 milligrams of chondroitin sulfates. Between 120 and 200 pounds: 1,500 milligrams of glucosamine and 1,200 milligrams of chondroitin sulfates. More than 200 pounds, 2,000 milligrams of glucosamine plus 1,600 milligrams of chondroitin sulfates." He suggests dividing the glucosamine and chondroitin supplements into two to four doses, taken throughout the day with food. He and other experts also advise adjusting the dose to fit your individual response. Some people get better right away and cut their initial doses by one-half to one-third, says Dr. Theodosakis. People who are obese or on diuretics may need higher doses, some European studies suggest.

How Quickly Does It Work?
Some people feel a little better within a week or two. Generally, improvement should be noticeable within eight

weeks. However, it's important to understand that although relief of pain and other symptoms may be almost immediate, true rebuilding of body cartilage, addressing the underlying cause of the disease, takes time. Thus the longer the use, the greater the benefits. Glucosamine is classified as a "slow-acting drug" in Germany. The idea is twofold: to control symptoms in a few days or weeks, thus avoiding or diminishing the use of strong painkillers, and to stop or reduce degeneration of cartilage degenerative process over the long-term treatment.

What Can You Expect?

Not everyone with osteoarthritis improves after taking glucosamine-chondroitin agents, and the remedy is not guaranteed to make you pain-free or totally mobile. However, many people do respond dramatically, being able to reduce or eliminate NSAIDS and other painkillers and postpone or avoid joint replacement surgery. You can hasten your progress by also having a program of regular exercise (more likely when pain is less), losing excessive weight, and eating a good diet, including fish high in omega–3 fatty acids.

The earlier you start using glucosamine, the better. Studies show it is very effective for early or less severe osteoarthritis, but less so for severe or late osteoarthritis. The reason: When there is little or no cartilage left on joints, it cannot be regenerated or repaired.

The Safety Factor

Side effects are minimal or nonexistent. In the large Portuguese study, about 12 percent of the subjects registered complaints from glucosamine, mostly mild to moderate gastrointestinal upset, including heartburn, nausea, gastric pain, and dyspepsia. As for long-term toxicity, animal studies by an Italian team of researchers pronounced glu-cosamine at least 1,000 to 4,000 times safer than indo-methacin, a common NSAID prescribed for osteoarthritis. Feeding small lab animals as much as one-third of a pound of glucosamine every day for over a year produced no toxicity. If you are pregnant, check with your physician before using glucosamine. It's best to take the supple-ments with food, especially if you have a peptic ulcer or have an upset stomach after taking it.

CAN YOU TAKE IT WITH OTHER DRUGS?
Apparently, glucosamine does not interfere with the activ-ity of NSAIDS, aspirin, or other ant-iinflammatory or analgesic medications. Some animal evidence, in fact, suggests glucosamine may protect cartilage against that long-term damage from anti-inflammatory agents. Adding glucosamine may allow you to reduce doses of anti-inflammatory drugs or stop taking them altogether.

What's the Alternative?
The mainstay of arthritis drug treatment in the United States is a family of medicines known as nonsteroidal anti-inflammatory drugs (NSAIDS), including aspirin and ibuprofen. Sadly, they can be quite harmful. Their use to treat arthritis has created an epidemic of bleeding ulcers, says Dr. James F. Fries, Stanford University medical pro-fessor and arthritis expert. NSAIDS account for 10,000 to 20,000 deaths and 100,000 to 200,000 hospitalizations each year, he says. About one-fourth of those who use NSAIDS to relieve chronic pain develop ulcers.

Consumer Concerns
You can buy glucosamine and chondroitin sulfates sepa-rately in varying strengths under numerous brands in

health food stores, pharmacies and other retail outlets. Glucosamine is more readily available than chondroitin. Although Dr. Theodosakis insists that all forms of glucosamine (sulfate, hydrocholoride, n-acetyl, chlorhydrate, D-glucosamine) are essentially the same, another expert on glucosamines, Michael Murray, N.D., of Seattle, vigorously disagrees. Dr. Murray points out that nearly all the European research demonstrating success in treating osteoarthritis has used glucosamine sulfate alone, not other forms of glucosamine and not in combination with chondroitins. He says there is no clinical evidence showing that taking glucosamine with chondroitin is superior to taking glucosamine sulfate alone.

The brand-name suuplement used by the two people cited in this chapter—Phyllis Eagelton and Mollie Hauck—which is also the brand being tested by Dr. Das in his new research, is a combination of glucosamine and chondroitin known as Cosamin DS (Double Strength) made by the Nutramax Company in Baltimore. Each pill contains 500 milligrams of glucosamine chlorhydrate, 400 milligrams of chondroitin sulfate, as well as 66 milligrams of vitamin C and 10 milligrams of manganese. Licensed health professionals can obtain it by calling 800-925-5187. Consumers can call the same number to get the name of a local or mail-order dispensing pharmacy that sells the product. A similar combination glucosamine HCl-chondroitin sulfate supplement is also being sold directly to consumers as Osteo-Bi-Flex 450 from Sundown and GlucoPro 900 from Thompson Nutritional Products.

Should You Try It?
Absolutely. Glucosamine should be the "remedy of choice" for osteoarthritis, the first thing to try. It may relieve pain and enable you to delay or avoid joint replacement

surgery. If it doesn't work, you will find out in a couple of months with no harm done, since side effects are minimal.

Which Type Should You Take?

It seems likely that glucosamine sulfate alone (as proved by many well-designed studies), or a combination of glucosamine and chodroitins, including Cosamin, (as many case histories support) may all work. The only way to really find out which works best for you is to do some trial-and-error experimenting; test them yourself and go with the one or ones that give the most relief.

Will It Work for Other Forms of Arthritis?

Perhaps. Pharmacist Robert Henderson, the developer of Cosamin and president of Nutramax, says his glucosamine product was successful in recent tests on rat models for rheumatoid arthritis. Only one animal of twenty-four on Cosamin developed autoimmune dysfunction leading to rheumatoid-type arthritis, compared with more than half of the animals not given Cosamin, he says. Theoretically glucosamine-chondroitins should help stop cartilage destruction in rheumatoid arthritis as well as in osteo-arthritis, says Dr. Henderson. Studies need to be done to find out, but there are a few cases of success in juvenile arthritis.

MOLLIE'S MIRACLE
"If It Cures Racehorses, Why Not Me?"

When three-year-old Mollie woke up with a high fever, her parents, Kathy and Sam Hauck, thought it was a virus that would quickly disappear. It didn't. She became so sick she "could not move at all; she was totally immobilized," says her mother. Within a few weeks she was in intensive care at their hometown hospital in Oregon, fighting for her life. "She was slipping away; she was in so much pain, her body was shutting down. We were sure we were going to lose her." And nobody could say what was killing her.

Frantic, her parents got Mollie to another hospital, where she was diagnosed with juvenile rheumatoid arthritis and immediately put on corticosteroids (prednisone). In ten days they knew she was going to live. That was four years ago, and at age seven Mollie is still in pain. But her parents say she was much more crippled before she started taking an unusual antiarthritis pill usually reserved for animals, notably racehorses.

It is a substance the body makes naturally—glucosamine and chondroitins. Mollie's godfather, a veterinarian, was worried that Mollie's high doses of steroids over time would destroy her immune system. He suggested: Why not try nature's glucosamine, which he had found successful in treating animals with arthritis? Mollie started taking a large white capsule—literally a "horse pill" that her parents emptied and dissolved in apple juice or Kool-Aid.

Two years later she still takes it, because her parents say it has relieved her pain, made her more mobile, and dramatically improved her immune functioning. She's no longer a sitting duck for all the colds and flu and other infections she used to have, they say. Further, she is no longer confined to her wheelchair; now she just uses it when she becomes tired or has a bad day of pain in her feet.

"Before she got on Cosamin, we constantly carried Mollie everywhere, carried her in and out of bed, carried her shopping; but we no longer have to do that," says her mother. "It maintains Mollie so she can move and function on a day-to-day basis. She is not in pain twenty-four hours a day where she can't move like she was before.

"It just blew me away to find out we've used this stuff for years on animals to keep them healthy and arthritis pain-free, but not given it to humans. It's scary. Of course, you can't just go into a vet's office and say give me some of that stuff you give horses for my arthritis. But if it works, why not?"

Mollie still takes conventional medicines, but her parents hope eventually to drop them because they fear the long-term side effects. "It's sad our society relies on so many drugs," says Kathy Hauck. As far as anyone knows, Mollie was the first child to try this form of glucosamine. Since then Dr. Henderson has heard of similar successes in other cases of juvenile arthritis, but no controlled studies have been done to confirm the efficacy.

What Else Is It Good For?
You could try glucosamine for virtually any type of joint pain or injury, says biochemist Luke R. Bucci, Ph.D., an authority on glucosamines and the author of *Pain-Free: The Definitive Guide to Healing Arthritis, Low-Back Pain, and Sports Injuries Through Nutrition and Supplements*, the first book on the topic. Dr. Bucci says the supplements should help treat "any conditions that involve repair of cartilage and joints . . . including osteoarthritis, rheumatoid arthritis, ankylosing spondylitis, invertebral disc con-

ditions, chondromalacia [a softening of the kneecap], tendinitis, bursitis, postsurgical repair of traumatic injury to joints, traumatic injury to joints, and tenosynovitis." He speculates that glucosamine would also be therapeutic in repairing fractures, torn tendons, and ligaments.

Unique
Infection Fighter

(E C H I N A C E A)

It's America's most popular herbal medicine, against colds, flu, viruses, infections of all kinds. If you want to know why 30 million Americans take it, and German researchers praise it, give it a try yourself.

If you're hit by a cold or another bacterial infection, you can fight it by drowning in a sea of antibiotics that are fast becoming worthless because bacteria develop a tolerance for them. Or if the culprit is a virus, you are virtually helpless because our best pharmaceutical minds have not been able to come up with antiviral agents that are effective, even against the common cold. Isn't it time to try a different approach—attempting to fortify ourselves against the pathological invaders so they are less able to make us sick and kill us? Certainly many scientists are working on drugs or immunostimulants designed to bolster our natural defenses against infectious agents, as well as cancer. But one such natural remedy is already in widespread use; it's easily obtainable; it's inexpensive; and if it doesn't manage to chase your infection away, at least it will not harm you while trying.

What makes echinacea unique is that it does not mimic the magic bullets of conventional medicine. Here's the difference: If you have an infection, you can try to cure it by taking something to do three things: curtail the symptoms; disable or destroy the particular microorganism causing the infection; or boost your general immune defenses, overwhelming the infectious agents so the symptoms eventually go away. In a cold, for example, decongestants may reduce the sniffles but not thwart the underlying disease. Typical antibiotics can kill the actual bacteria that cause a disease such as pneumonia. On the other hand, a drug like interferon can stimulate the body to marshal an army of soldiers, such as antibodies and pathogen-eating macrophages, raising general resistance to various nonspecific infectious agents. It's sort of like fending off enemies by shooting bullets to kill them or making yourself more resistant to their attacks by cloaking yourself in armor that wards off all attacks from everywhere.

If you want to activate your immune system as a way of defeating infections (as well as other diseases that flourish on lowered immunity, such as cancer), the "remedy of choice"—the first thing to try—is echinacea. Echinacea has made its medical mark, notably in European studies, as an "immunostimulant" to strengthen the body against infectious agents of all sorts, whether viruses or bacteria. Echinacea does not directly kill or disable infectious bacteria. However, recent research suggests echinacea does directly attack viruses, making it a rarity among remedies of all types, including pharmaceuticals. Echinacea is most often used as a remedy against the common cold and flu, but it looks promising against a broad array of pathogens. It is the number one best-selling herbal remedy in health food stores in the United

States, with sales up 25 percent in 1996. And millions say it works, sometimes when all else fails.

GAYLE'S MIRACLE
"At Last, My Mysterious Virus Was Gone"

It was an ordeal that Gayle Carter, a twenty-nine-year-old editor for Gannett's Sunday magazine supplement, *USA Weekend*, recalls with almost perfect clarity. In March 1996 she thought she had the flu. But it lasted for weeks. "I just couldn't shake it." One doctor gave her antibiotics. But she got worse. "I started to have this incredible neck and ear pain." Thinking she had an ear infection, she consulted an ear, nose, and throat specialist. At the time her fever was "a raging 102." She would wake up sweating. The new doctor blamed "some sort of virus," either mono or Epstein-Barr, and sent her home to "rest and let it run its course." The pain in the right side of her neck was so intense that she could barely sleep. Not even a prescription of super-strength Motrin helped. After eight weeks she was still running a fever of about 100, had a horrendous sore throat, and suffered pain throughout her body—even the soles of her feet hurt. She went to an infectious disease specialist who, alarmed at the neck pain, ordered an MRI to be sure it was not a tumor.

Then she heard about the herb echinacea from some new acquaintances. "I bought an herb book, looked it up, bought some, and started to take it. My fever broke after one week on it—two pills a day, each 400 milligrams, for a total of 800 milligrams."

She was elated. Her bad sore throat started to disappear also. She skipped echinacea for a few days and the fever returned. "So I went back on it and the fever went away, she says. "As soon as I started taking it, I began to feel good again."

With the high fever and sore throat mostly gone, she could function again. "At last, I could go on living." But she was still in some pain. She had also been diagnosed with fibromyalgia, a form of arthritis, possibly related to her chronic Epstein-Barr viral infection. In July 1996, she went to see James Gordon, M.D., a clinical professor at the Georgetown University School of Medicine and director of the Center for Mind-Body Medicine in Washington. He recommended she continue on echinacea for three to four weeks to help fight the virus and stimulate her immunity. Additionally, he advised taking daily 3,000 milligrams of vitamin C; a multivitamin mineral tablet; many herbs, including astragalus, red peony, and licorice. He also recommended acupuncture, yoga, and physical manipulations of her neck and upper back to relieve pain. Dr. Gordon attributed much of her jaw and neck pain to fibromyalgia, but some also was due to misalignment of vertebra from minor injuries in an automobile accident. The pain gradually went away and the suffering patient returned to normal good health.

Gayle is sold on echinacea. "It really helped save me over and over. I know it boosts my immune system." Dr. Gordon agrees. "The echinacea certainly seemed to have helped her, which is no surprise, because research shows it is antiviral and enhances immunity. I take it myself if I feel the symptoms of a cold or flu coming on." However, he stresses that echinacea, albeit effective, is not a magic bullet for chronic conditions such as fibromyalgia. "You need a comprehensive, integrated approach," he says, "that addresses the complex multiple underlying causes, not just symptoms." Unfortunately, doctors relying exclusively on Western conventional medicine tend to treat individual symptoms and miss the big picture, says Dr. Gordon.

During her four-month search for relief, Gayle Carter saw twelve medical doctors—four internists; two ear, nose, and throat specialists; three infectious disease specialists; one rheumatologist; a radiologist; and, at last, Dr. Gordon.

What Is It?

Echinacea (pronounced ek-in-NAY-sha) also known as purple coneflower, is a native American plant. It was introduced into medical practice in the United States in 1887 and used extensively to treat minor infections, such as cold and flu, for about four decades. In 1938 a German pharmaceutical company began scientific research on the American plant, developing a medicinal product that engendered worldwide interest in the herb. Most of the scientific testing of the herb has been done in Germany, where it is officially approved as an over-the-counter drug to boost immunity and help fight respiratory infections and urinary tract infections.

What's the Evidence?

Echinacea fights infections by boosting immune functioning, says Dr. Varro Tyler, a leading authority on medicinal plants and dean emeritus of the School of Pharmacy at

Purdue University. He points to recent German studies. For example, in 1992 two well-conducted German studies concluded that echinacea helped people get over colds and flu faster and reduced their severity. The plant worked especially well on people with weakened immune systems. One study tested echinacea on 108 people, ages thirteen to eighty-four, who were prone to infections—they had suffered at least three cold-connected infections the previous winter. For eight weeks, half the group got 4 milliliters twice a day of echinacea purpurea juice (Echinacin Liquidum); the other half got an inactive extract or placebo. The results: The echinacea takers cut their chances of getting a cold by 36 percent. Additionally, their colds were usually "mild." The echinacea takers had one-third fewer "moderate to severe" cold symptoms. Researchers concluded that, when subjected to the most rigorous standards, echinacea boosted immunity, preventing colds and cutting their duration. Further, most apt to benefit were the most vulnerable—those with "inferior immune systems" as indicated by low blood levels of specific infection-fighting T cells.

In a similar German study of 180 normal, healthy volunteers, ages eighteen to sixty, echinacea cut episodes of flu short and reduced upper respiratory flu symptoms. Important in this study was the proper dose, which was higher than usual. Echinacea was no better than a dummy pill at a lower dose of two daily droppersful (90 drops or 450 milligrams). But a daily dose of four droppersful (180 drops or 900 milligrams) produced "good or very good," results, supervising doctors said, reducing overall flu symptoms dramatically in three or four days. Signs of flu, such as stuffy nose, sneezing, chills, weakness, sore throat, headaches, and muscle pains, declined by 75 percent in the echinacea takers, compared with 37 percent in those on the inactive placebo. In other words, echinacea was about twice as effective as a "sugar pill" in fighting the flu.

THE GERMANS GIVE IT THUMBS UP
One way scientists get an overall scientific fix on a medicine is to examine all the human studies ever done on the substance—old studies, new studies, studies that are less rigorous in design, and studies that meet the highest standards of modern testing. That's what a German team of researchers led by Professor Hildebert Wagner at the University of Munich did regarding echinacea in 1994. They found twenty-six controlled trials; not surprisingly, most of the older studies were of "modest" quality. But Dr. Wagner concluded that several more recent studies clearly established the immune-stimulating and infection-fighting benefits of echinacea alone or combined with other herbs. Echinacea proved effective in preventing and treating upper respiratory tract infections, such as colds, according to three good studies. The best study of echinacea alone supported the strong dose of 900 milligrams daily. The widely acclaimed use of echinacea to stimulate immune functioning is scientifically valid, Dr. Wagner concluded, but he said the best type and dose were still unclear.

How Does It Work?
Reportedly, echinacea fends off infections primarily by activating immune functions and, secondarily, by attacking viruses. Exactly how it accomplishes this and what agents in the herb trigger the flood of increased immune activity are still unclear, although several herb constituents have demonstrated antiviral and immune-potentiating activity in dozens of laboratory studies against a variety of infectious agents, including influenza, herpes, and polio.

The University of Munich's Dr. Wagner theorizes that echinacea boosts immune functions by prodding stem cells in bone marrow and lymphatic tissue to produce stronger and greater numbers of white cells, including T-lymphocytes, to fight infections. In one study, echinacea boosted T-lymphocyte activity 20 to 30 percent more than an agent specifically designed to boost such activity. In another study, echinacea caused certain infection-fighting white cells—leukocytes—to rise faster in people with exclusively viral infections than in those with predominantly bacterial infections, indicating that echinacea is better at fighting viral infections than bacterial infections.

Another exciting explanation: Echinacea stimulates production of interferon, a natural body substance of momentous importance in the body's overall defense system. Specifically, interferon activates natural killer cells, inciting them to attach to cells infected with viruses or to tumor cells, causing them to disintegrate. Further, interferon triggers release of enzymes that disrupt the genetic machinery (DNA) of viruses, blocking their ability to replicate and spread. If the virus can't reproduce, the infection is stopped or short-lived. Thus echinacea appears to possess the added power of stopping viruses. Certainly any agent that can boost interferon is big-time. Synthetic interferon, you may remember, has been seriously studied as a way of boosting the immune system to fight off cancer.

BABY MATTHEW'S MIRACLE
The Antibiotic Alternative

Like many two-year-olds, Matthew Saunders* developed an ear infection, known as otitis media. The standard treatment is antibiotics. If that fails, doctors typically insert tiny tubes into the youngsters' ears to drain them. It's expensive and has virtually no long-term benefits. But fortunately, Matthew never got either. His pediatrician is Jay Gordon, M.D., at Cedars Sinai Medical Center, who also is a clinical instructor at UCLA Medical Center. (Dr. Jay Gordon is not related to Dr. James Gordon, mentioned previously.) Little Matthew instead got 5 to 10 drops of echinacea three times a day in a glass of juice. His ear infection cleared up within two or three days. Further, Matthew also stopped getting colds, coughs, and runny nose and other infections.

For about fifteen years Dr. Gordon has been using the herb echinacea as first-line treatment for common ear infections in infants and children, with great success. "I have treated many hundreds, perhaps thousands of cases of ear infections with echinacea, and I know it works. I rarely have to give antibiotics or use tubes to clear up these infections," he says. Although Dr. Gordon has not kept statistical records or done controlled studies, he estimates echinacea helps clear up ear infections in most cases, making it far more effective and economical than conventional solutions of drugs and tubes. He says it does not cure every case, nor does it always eliminate the need for antibiotics, but it helps in every case by boosting immune functioning. Dr. Gordon also uses echinacea to fight all kinds of infections in infants and youngsters, including colds and flu. He usually advises alternating taking the herb for two weeks, then stopping for two weeks, and so on for as long as necessary.

*A pseudonym has been used to protect privacy, but the medical details are accurate.

How Much Do You Need?

Since echinacea comes in different forms, from the flower or root and as liquid or solid, recommended dosages vary. Thus check the product's label for proper doses. In general, however, to fight a cold, flu, or other infections, adults generally need 900 milligrams a day of solid dry powdered standardized extract, say experts. Take it in doses of 300 milligrams three times daily. For children under age six, Seattle's Dr. Donald Brown recommends half the adult dosage.

At the first signs of cold or flu, Dr. Brown advises taking echinacea for ten to fourteen days without interrution.

The Safety Factor

Echinacea may cause mild side effects, such as stomach upset and diarrhea. there are no reports of toxicity from taking it. Experts warn against using echinacea if you have an autoimmune disease, such as lupus, or other progressive systematic illnesses such as tuberculosis, multiple sclerosis, diabetes, and in particular AIDS. (There's evidence echinacea may even promote HIV infections). Also don't take echinacea if you are allergic to flowers of the daisy family, cautions Dr. Brown.

Commission E also recommends not taking echinacea for more than eight weeks without interruption. However, this is not because of any evidence of harm from such continual use; nor does echinacea lose its effectiveness from constant use. Commission E was simply expressing the general principle that you shouldn't take any remedy if you don't really need it, according to Dr. Varro Tyler.

Should You Try It?

Yes, particularly for colds and flu and acute respiratory infections, preferably in the early stages. If you feel a cold or the flu coming on, you may want to take echinacea every day for about two weeks or until symptoms disappear. Echinacea may also help fight off other viral and bacterial infections, such as strep throat, staph infections, recurring vaginal yeast infections, urinary tract infections, herpes, bronchitis, and ear infections.

Caution: Although it's okay to treat common colds and flu with echinacea, self-diagnosing and self-treating chronic infections with echinacea could be unwise. Such infections may have an underlying and perhaps reversible cause and need medical attention. It's best to discuss the use of echinacea with a health professional and seek medical advice if symptoms of an infection don't disappear after a couple of weeks of using echinacea.

KERRY'S MIRACLE
"The Child's Infections Disappeared"

Can you use echinacea continuously to prevent infections that may crop up or to keep chronic infections under control? Although you often hear that you should cycle echinacea, taking it for a time, then stopping before taking it again, many experts say it's perfectly safe and effective to take continuously. International authority Kerry Bone, a practitioner of herbal medicine and a founder of MediHerb, Australia's largest herbal medicine manufacturer, says he and many Australians "take it for long periods of time as a general immune herb, and it's just so effective."

To illustrate, he recounts a case of a three-year-old girl brought to him by her despairing mother. "The mother was crying and at her wit's end; her little girl was so susceptible to infections she had had twenty-five courses of antibiotics by the age of three! She had nearly constant lower and upper respiratory infections, colds, and bronchitis, and she was asthmatic." After treating the symptoms of the bronchitis, Bone put the child on daily echinacea. "For the whole year that I saw her, she never had another infection," he says. "When herbs do things like that, word gets around." To her mother, it was a miracle.

In Bone's view, this case epitomizes the difference between herbal and conventional medicines. "Herbal medicine aims at the basic cause of the problem, not just superficial symptoms," he says. "A physician may give an antibiotic that clears up an infection, but it doesn't stop the next one, because your immune system is not working properly. Someone using herbs tries to correct the weakened immunity so the infection does not recur."

Dr. Luke Bucci, an American authority on herbal medicines, agrees that "cycling echinacea is a dogma with no scientific support. I think it's okay to use it all the time as an immune-stimulant if needed," he says.

Consumer Concerns

Various brands and types of echinacea are sold in the United States. Echinacea comes as a tincture, tablet, and capsule, and even in flavors for children. The best tested and most extensively used worldwide is a product called Echinacin in Germany. It is imported and sold in the United States under the brand name EchinaGuard by Nature's Way.

God's Valium

(VALERIAN)

It's a splendid sleeping pill and a fix for anxiety, and it doesn't make you feel bad later. What more could you ask?

Would you like a good night's sleep without the morning hangover from sleeping pills? Or a cure for anxiety without the overkill of high-potency sedative drugs? Or a muscle relaxant that does not have the side effects of Valium? Valerian, a natural mild herbal sedative, could be a solution. About 40 million Americans have chronic sleep disorders, and 30 million others have occasional problems falling and staying asleep. Sales of prescription sedatives and tranquilizers, such as Valium and Halcion, are astronomical—about 10 million people take them every year, mainly to cure sleep troubles. The medications have frightening side effects, including a risk of addiction or overdose, and withdrawal problems. Halcion has caused horrendous side effects in some users, including psychotic disturbances, memory loss, and hallucinations. So profound is the problem that it makes one wonder why someone cannot come up with a good, safe, gentle sleeping pill.

Well, someone did eons ago, and millions of people already know about it and use it. The herb valerian tranquilizes safely and gently without a risk of addiction, and is widely used and approved in other countries as an alternative to our potent, dangerous sedative drugs. Some call it "God's Valium." And there's plenty of evidence that it works to calm you down, tame the brain, reduce anxiety, induce sleep, relieve stress, and even relax muscles without a morning hangover or permanent harm. So in a choice between human-made Valium and "God's Valium" (valerian), you may want to give the ancient version, backed by thousands of years of human use, a chance before opting for the upstart imitations.

DR. BROWN'S MIRACLE
"Valerian Cured His Anxiety and Got Him off Xanax"

Dr. Donald J. Brown is a nationally renowned naturopathic doctor who teaches at Bastyr University in Seattle and often lectures to physicians at medical schools on the science of natural remedies. He is the author of several books, including *Herbal Prescriptions for Better Health*. One natural substance Dr. Brown talks about often is valerian. He is a big fan of the natural antianxiety agent and recommends it to patients as the number one remedy for sleeping problems. "It's much better and safer than, say, melatonin." Dr. Brown likes to tell other doctors about his enormous success using valerian to treat anxiety and panic attacks, especially in helping patients withdraw from prescription antianxiety drugs such as Xanax.

He tells of one case—a thirty-four-year-old male jazz musician who started taking Xanax to relieve his anxiety, especially when he was on tour. To quell the panic attacks, which became worse when he had to fly long distances on planes, he had been taking Xanax in fairly heavy doses for about a year and a half. Twice he had tried to stop the Xanax because he feared he was getting addicted. To wean himself off it, he dropped his Xanax dosage as low as 0.5 milligram a day. But when he quit entirely, he seemed to have a "rebound" effect. The anxiety and panic attacks returned with a vengeance, seemingly worse than before; his anxiety was so debilitating that he could no longer travel. To survive, he had to go back on Xanax. Discouraged and concerned, he consulted Dr. Brown, who suggested that he start taking valerian while gradually reducing the dose of Xanax. After about five weeks the musician stopped taking Xanax altogether but stayed on Valerian. To his great relief the anxiety and panic attacks did not return. He was able to cope perfectly well on valerian alone. And when he decided to stop taking it routinely he had no symptoms of withdrawal. He now takes valerian only occasionally to prevent an attack of anxiety when he is in a precarious situation, such as having to fly.

How is valerian able to conduct such a smooth withdrawal? Dr. Brown speculates it's because the herbal medicine binds to the same receptor sites on brain cells as Xanax. When Xanax goes away, the receptors "scream out for something to bind to," he says. If there's nothing there, they go nuts. But if you can slip in valerian, it's enough to satisfy them so they calm down. Dr. Brown says many doctors are now using valerian to help ensure a safe, calm passage away from the torments of Xanax.

What Is It?

The root of valerian, a tall, fernlike plant, has served for thousands of years as a mild sedative. From 1820 until 1942 valerian was listed in the U.S. Pharmacopoeia as a tranquilizer. It's widely used and approved in Europe as a mild hypnotic to induce sleep and relieve anxiety. More than 5 million units of valerian are sold in Germany and about 10 million in France every year. In the United Kingdom valerian is also a popular and government-approved sleep aid. It is also approved in Belgium, Switzerland, and Italy as an over-the-counter medication for insomnia.

What's the Evidence?

Of all plant sedatives, valerian appears most effective, says medicinal plant expert Dr. Varro Tyler. So convincing is the evidence of valerian's efficacy and safety that a coalition of European manufacturers of phytomedicines (plant medicines) have petitioned the FDA to allow claims for valerian as an over-the-counter nighttime sleeping "aid," defined as an agent that relaxes and mildly sedates. More than 200 scientific studies on the pharmacology of valerian have been published in the scientific literature, mostly in Europe in the last thirty years.

Valerian is a well-tested sleeping potion. At least six controlled clinical trials in Europe show that valerian can shorten the time to fall asleep, prolong sleep time, increase deep sleep stages, increase dreaming, reduce nighttime awakenings, and significantly improve the quality of sleep in both normal sleepers and insomniacs. Classic is the study of 128 volunteers at the Nestlé Research Laboratories in Switzerland in the mid-1980s; for three nights at a time they took either valerian extract or a sugar pill. Valerian won out; 37 percent on valerian said they fell asleep faster, compared with 23 percent on placebo. Further, 43 percent said they slept better versus 25 percent on placebo. Even 45 percent of good sleepers said they "slept better than usual" on valerian. But habitually bad sleepers got the most benefit. The same was true in a double-blind Swedish test. Forty-four percent of poor sleepers said they had "perfect sleep" after taking a product with 400 milligrams of valerian. Eighty-nine percent said their sleep improved.

VALERIAN OR HALCION?

Valerian even equaled the powerful drug Halcion as a sleeping pill. A 1992 German study compared a combination valerian pill (160 milligrams of valerian and 80 milligrams lemon balm) with Halcion (0.125 milligrams triazolam) in twenty people, ages thirty to fifty. Over a period of nine nights, the valerian combination put subjects to sleep just as fast and produced the same sound sleep as Halcion. It was most effective in so-called bad sleepers. However, unlike the valerian takers, the Halcion users suffered hangovers and loss of concentration the next day.

Virtually all tests clearly pinpoint the big difference between valerian and prescription drugs, such as Valium and Halcion. The herb does not produce morning hangovers of drowsiness, reduction in concentration, and impaired physical performance. Nor does it interact with alcohol to accentuate impairment as do prescription drugs. A 1995 German study found no interaction between alcohol and valerian that lessened concentration, attentiveness, reaction time, or performance in driving a car. In short, valerian is okay to take when you are awake and active, as well as when you are going to sleep, making it much more desirable, especially in cases when a person simply wants to put a mild damper on anxiety or stress during the day.

Nevertheless, experts also point out that valerian has many fewer side effects precisely because it does not hit your brain with a hammer the way many prescription drugs do. In other words, valerian is much milder. "Valerian and plant drugs do not have the degree of activity of prescription drugs, nor do they have the drawbacks," says authority Dr. Varro Tyler.

How Does It Work?

The mechanism of valerian in the brain appears similar to that of the benzodiazepine drugs—Halcion and Valium. These tend to sedate by stimulating activity of the nerve transmitter GABA (gamma-aminobutyric acid), which dampens the brain's arousal system. In animals, valerian does the same thing, triggering release of GABA from the brain cortex. In mice, both valerian and Valium prolong sleep. Research at the Institute of Pharmaceutical Biology in Marburg, Germany, showed that sedating constituents in valerian can bind to the same receptor sites on brain cells as barbiturates and benzodiazepines. In fact, valerian bounced benzodiazepines off the receptor sites of animal brain cells.

Which constituents in valerian sedate the central nervous system is still a matter of dispute. Several have been identified, including valerenic acid and valepotriates, chemicals unique to valerian. Valerenic acid is a prime constituent in European products and is often combined with other mildly sedating herbs, such as lemon balm, passion flower, and chamomile. According to naturalist Stephen Foster, more than 120 active chemicals have been detected in valerian. Foster suggests that a combination of valerian's compounds work together synergistically to promote sedation.

Who Should Take It?

You can use valerian as a remedy to help you relax, sleep better, calm down in moments of mild anxiety and stress—even before giving a speech or before getting on an airplane if you are afraid to fly—or as a muscle relaxant. You can take it during the day or at night for sleep. Valerian can also ease the symptoms of withdrawing from Xanax, Valium, and other benzodiazepines and can serve as a substitute for these drugs in people with mild to moderate anxiety and insomnia.

DR. DANE'S MIRACLE
A Quick Fix Without Pain

Skip Dane, a professor in the health sciences department of Brigham Young University, with a Ph.D. from the University of Chicago, lifted the 650-pound weight off the rack, put it on his shoulders, squatted down, and began to stand back up. Two years before, on his fiftieth birthday, he had set a record for squats at the university and since then had broken it by doing a squat with 800 pounds on his shoulders. But on that evening in 1995, as he started to stand up, he could feel the quadriceps muscle in his left thigh give out. He rolled back and dropped the weight. The pain in his thigh was excruciating. "It really hurt," he recalls. He managed to stretch the muscle enough to hobble around and get home. He made it through the night without painkillers.

Dane, a champion weight-lifter who does research on "hardiness training" at the university, knew that ordinarily an injury like that would take three or four weeks to heal if treated with typical painkillers. But the treatment recommended by his doctor, Dennis Remington, M.D., was not pain-killers. A medical doctor who also has training in naturopathic medicine, Remington prescribed valerian root along with saw palmetto and a massage. "I was back to doing squats at 600 in six days," marvels Dane. The valerian, he says, acted as a muscle relaxant, relieving the pain, and the saw palmetto accelerated the healing process by reducing inflammation. "If you've got an injured muscle and you can totally relax it and reduce the swelling, the healing process is going to be much accelerated," says Dr. Dane. That's what the two herbal remedies did. During the six-day interim, he was even able to continue working out with a bench press, but he did not do squats or leg presses.

The total cost of the treatment: $10. Dr. Dane and his family are insured by American West Life Insurance, one of the few health plans that regularly cover herbal remedies.

How Much Do You Need?

Start out with a low dose and, if needed, work up to a higher dose. For use as a sleeping pill, Dr. Donald Brown recommends taking 300 to 500 milligrams of a standardized valerian extract about an hour before bedtime. Cut that dose in half when taking valerian as a mild tranquilizer to quiet anxiety during the day, he says. One hundred fifty to 300 milligrams translates into one-half to one teaspoonful as a fluid extract, and one to one and a half teaspoons as a tincture. You should notice effects within thirty to forty-five minutes.

The Safety Factor

Side effects at recommended doses are minor. Most common is occasional stomach upset. However, in large doses valerian could cause headache, restlessness, nausea, and morning grogginess. (If you are sleepy or groggy the next morning, the dosage may be too high for you; simply reduce the amount you are taking, experts advise.) Valerian, unlike prescription sleeping pills, is not addictive or a cause of any mental disturbances. There are no reports in animals or humans of serious poisoning or death from overdoses of valerian. However, some clinicians have noted that some individuals have an idiosyncratic (opposite to what is expected) response to valerian; they become more excited and revved up instead of relaxed and calm.

In the only known case of an overdose of valerian, a woman took forty to fifty capsules of powdered valerian root (Nature's Way Products, Inc., 470 milligrams each) in a suicide attempt. Half an hour later, she experienced fatigue, abdominal cramping, chest tightness, lightheadedness, and foot and hand tremor. She was back to normal within twenty-four hours. Doctors concluded that valerian, at an overdose of 20 grams (20,000 milligrams), is not acutely poisonous. The Food and Drug Administration lists valerian as GRAS (generally recognized as safe).

Caution: It's okay to use valerian on your own for mild anxiety and sleep problems. If you have serious anxiety or insomnia or have been diagnosed with or treated for psychiatric problems, or are taking other psychiatric drugs of any kind, consult your doctor before self-treating with valerian. Because of the possibility of withdrawal symptoms, switching from prescription drugs to valerian should be done under the supervision of a doctor.

Who Should Not Take It?

Valerian is not advised for pregnant or lactating women, children under age two, or in combination with other over-the-counter or prescription tranquilizers or sedatives.

Important: If you have chronic insomnia, you should also go easy on caffeine; high doses of caffeine can neutralize some of the sedating effects of valerian.

Consumer Concerns

Most of the European research has been done on standardized valerian products. To get this research-quality valerian, look for labels indicating water-soluble extracts "standardized" for valerenic acid content (0.8 percent valerenic acid).

Little Liver Pills That Really Work

(MILK THISTLE)

Whose liver needs help? Just about everybody's. Liver damage is a plague of modern life. Here's nature's way of curing it.

Pity your poor liver. All those awful poisons you take in must pass through this chemical factory of detoxification. If the toxins are more than your liver can handle, liver cells are destroyed, liver function can decline, and that incredibly important organ can eventually shut down. Even if, like most Americans, you don't worry much about your liver, you should. Your liver is burdened by the toxic offspring of modern civilization: environmental chemicals, air pollutants, pesticides, auto exhaust, prescription and nonprescription drugs, and alcohol, all of which can inflict severe unexpected liver injury. Indeed, alcohol causes 80 percent of all liver disease in Western countries. Even moderate drinkers frequently have a fatty liver, indicating incipient liver damage. And if your liver is damaged, you will find little hope for recovery in conventional mainstream medicine. The treatments of choice: powerful steroids and immunosuppressants, and, as a last resort, liver transplant.

That's why if you drink a little more alcohol than you should; or take drugs that can damage your liver, such as cholesterol-lowering medications, acetaminophen, and antidepressants; or use pesticides; or work around industrial chemicals such as carbon tetrachloride; or already have signs of impaired liver function, you should know about the marvelous seeds of a special plant called *Silybum marianum,* or milk thistle. This herb is nature's answer to modern life's constant bombardment of the body by toxic substances.

In Europe, where the liver gets more attention and respect and people vigorously guard the liver with tonics and treatments, milk thistle is a popular botanical liver medicine supported by solid scientific evidence showing it can prevent and reverse liver damage, regenerating cells and large areas of liver tissue. Most of the research has been done in Germany, where the herb is government-endorsed as a supportive treatment for chronic inflammatory liver conditions and cirrhosis.

Milk thistle deserves serious attention as a way to forestall a liver catastrophe brought on by the perils of modern life. The herb could be your best hope for a miracle cure or for avoiding the need for a miracle cure.

What Is It?

Milk thistle, as its name implies, is a weed, a thistle topped by a prickly purplish flower containing seeds, packed with potent pharmacological benefits to the liver. It has been long heralded as a liver medicine; Pliny, the first-century Roman naturalist, recommended it, as did doctors in the Middle Ages and well into the nineteenth century. It fell largely out of favor in the twentieth century, until its recent revival, thanks to groundbreaking research in Germany.

What's the Evidence?

In the 1970s German researchers at the University of Munich validated milk thistle's long reputation as a hepatic folk medicine by identifying its liver-protecting pharmacological agents in the seeds or fruits of the flower and even detailing how they work against the most lethal liver toxins known. In a landmark series of studies, they showed that feeding rats a slow-acting liver-destroying chemical killed 100 percent of them in 130 days. But when animals simultaneously got milk thistle, 70 percent of them survived!

Since then, more than 200 experimental and clinical studies suggest that milk thistle is effective therapy for various liver diseases, including fatty liver—common in even moderate alcohol consumers—acute and chronic hepatitis, damage from drugs and exposure to toxic chemicals, and even advanced cirrhosis, which is usually irreversible and for which few pharmaceutical drugs do any good at all. One large-scale German study in 1992 reported phenomenal benefits from milk thistle in 2,637 patients with liver disorders, such as fatty liver, hepatitis, and cirrhosis. After eight weeks of taking standardized milk thistle capsules daily, 63 percent of the patients said their symptoms (nausea, fatigue, lack of appetite, abdominal distention) had disappeared. Lab tests confirmed that elevated liver enzymes, a sign of liver damage, had declined dramatically, as much as 46 percent. Further, 27 percent of enlarged livers had returned to normal size, and 56 percent had dramatically shrunk in size. Moreover, less than 1 percent of the milk thistle takers stopped taking the herb because of side effects, such as stomach upset, nausea, and light diarrhea.

REVERSING ALCOHOL DAMAGE

Milk thistle, fortunately, most strongly addresses the problem exactly where it is most needed. It does its best work in cells damaged by alcohol. According to research, it actually helps rebuild the ruined architecture of wounded liver cells, returning them to functional health. In one well-conducted (double-blind) study of 116 individuals with alcohol-induced liver damage, German researchers tested milk thistle in doses of 420 milligrams a day. The herb had a profound curative action within two weeks, as measured by favorable changes in enzymes, the markers of toxic liver cell damage. Indeed, investigators noticed improvement within seven days. Thus milk thistle helped restore normal liver function and curtail the course of the disease, researchers concluded. In another similarly high-quality study published in a German medical journal in 1981, investigators tested milk thistle in twenty-nine individuals with alcohol-induced liver disorders, including fatty liver, alcoholic hepatitis, and cirrhosis. The users improved significantly after two months on milk thistle, as shown by liver function tests. They also were much stronger, with better appetites and less nausea. In another investigation of fifty-seven patients with fatty liver, in those cases due to alcohol abuse, milk thistle depressed elevated GOT enzyme levels, a sign of liver damage, by 80 percent.

WHAT ABOUT HEPATITIS?

There's good evidence that milk thistle can help speed recovery in cases of hepatitis caused by a virus or alcohol. According to German research, milk thistle helped heal hepatitis B, the common form of hepatitis, most often resulting from a virus. It may also be successful in treating hepatitis C; studies to confirm it are under way. Considerable evidence shows that milk thistle helps in the treatment of chronic viral hepatitis. In a string of German studies, doctors gave patients with such hepatitis 420 milligrams of silymarin (milk thistle) daily for an average of nine months; it reversed liver injury, as measured by biopsy and decreased blood transaminase levels; transaminase is a liver enzyme that is elevated in hepatitis and is a primary marker of the intensity of the disease. Researchers deemed milk thistle effective for chronic hepatitis.

Italian investigators have also tested a relatively new milk thistle product, said to be particularly readily absorbed; silybin, the most highly active component of silymarin, is combined with another chemical, phosphatidylcholine, and is known as IdB 1016 or Silipide. In 1993 it was tested on sixty patients with either viral or alcohol-induced chronic hepatitis by researchers at the Institute of Clinical Medicine in Florence and produced remarkable decreases in enzymes resulting in greatly improved liver function. In a small test of eight older patients with chronic active hepatitis B and hepatitis C, the same milk thistle product improved liver function, as determined by enzyme levels, by 15 percent.

WILL IT WORK FOR CIRRHOSIS?
Milk thistle does not seem to reverse advanced cirrhosis in which symptoms are evident, such as ascites (abdominal accumulation of fluid) and esophageal or rectal bleeding. However, studies of excellent design (double-blind) have found that long-term use of milk thistle does slow down progression of the disease, which causes about 30,000 deaths in the United States annually. When taking milk thistle, cirrhotic patients are apt to survive longer, researchers have found, as illustrated by one large Ger-

man study in 1987 involving 170 patients with cirrhosis. For two years the patients got either 420 milligrams of silymarin a day or an inactive placebo pill. After two years the death rate of those getting the dummy pill was a striking 60 percent higher than that of those on milk thistle. The herb worked best in those with cirrhosis due to alcohol abuse.

Obviously milk thistle works best in cirrhosis when alcohol is eliminated. You can't continue to damage a weakened cirrhotic liver with alcohol and count on the herb to save you.

If you're taking pharmaceutical drugs, milk thistle may counter some of the drugs' ability to harm your liver. In an Italian test of sixty women in a hospital psychiatric ward, 400 milligrams of silymarin twice a day for three months softened the liver-damaging effects of the psychotropic drugs phenothiazines and butyrophenones, which they had been taking for at least five years. Milk thistle appears protective against the liver toxicity of acetaminophen or Tylenol. The analgesic in high doses can damage liver cells. According to Canadian and German studies in human cells, milk thistle blocks the drug's toxicity. In mice the herb has also inhibited damage from acetaminophen and the anticancer drug cisplatin.

There is good news for those who work around hazardous chemicals and breathe the vapors: Milk thistle helps protect against liver damage. About 25 percent of a group of 200 Hungarian workers in a chemical plant who had been exposed to toluene and xylene vapors for five to twenty years showed signs of liver damage. Some of them were given milk thistle for thirty days; others were not. Liver function tests found a definite improvement in the herb takers.

WHAT ABOUT CANCER?

Chronic inflammatory hepatitis is often a prelude to liver cancer, thus treating the inflammation, as milk thistle could, would be expected to help stop the development of cancer. Whether milk thistle can help treat liver cancer, a particularly difficult cancer, is unknown. Some people, as reported on the Internet, are using milk thistle to treat liver cancer, but no studies have been done to test its effectiveness.

The herb has protected mice from kidney and skin cancer. Incidentally, it has been noted that milk thistle stimulates regeneration of only healthy cells, not cancerous cells. Thus it would not be expected to encourage the spread of cancer. In Germany some doctors do recommend milk thistle to patients with liver cancer, believing it can do no harm and might help, especially in cases where mainstream medicine has little to offer.

THE CARPENTER'S MIRACLE
The Case of the Vanishing Liver Cancer

When the fifty-two-year-old German carpenter checked into a hospital at the University of Munich in July 1990, there was little doubt he had liver cancer. A CAT scan clearly showed a large tumor (measuring 4.5 centimeters) on the right lobe of his liver, and a biopsy confirmed extensive cancer in the right lobe, which had already spread to the left lobe. The man was a heavy drinker and smoker; he said he had drunk about 3 liters of beer every day for twenty years and smoked twenty cigarettes a day since adolescence. The team of treating physicians, including Mathis Grossmann, M.D., now at the University of Maryland Medical Biotechnology Center, deemed surgery useless because the cancer was so advanced. They discharged the patient, expecting him to die rather quickly. Patients with inoperable liver cancer typically survive only three to six months.

Thus the doctors were quite surprised when a year later, in June 1991, he showed up at the hospital again, looking much better. He had not smoked or drunk alcohol for a year, ever since the cancer was diagnosed, he said. He had gained 16 pounds and said he felt well. Most astonishing, the liver cancer had vanished. The physicians could find no trace of it. Ultrasound detected no tumor, and a CAT scan found only the footprints of a former cancer. Multiple biopsies of the tissue where the previous massive tumor was located found no malignancy. The cancer had totally regressed, shrunk, disappeared. Such spontaneous remission of any cancer is "a rare phenomenon," his doctors said, occurring only once in 60,000 to 100,000 patients. Only eight cases of complete regression of liver cancer have ever been published in the entire world medical literature, the doctors noted.

So what happened? What made the liver cancer go away? Was there anything unusual that prompted this "spontaneous remission"? The doctors were intrigued and perplexed, and offered this speculation: Maybe in some weird way the cancer starved to death. Or maybe the cessation of alcohol and smoking had something to do with recovery. But there is one other eventuality to be considered, they said: Right after the victim left the hospital with his incurable liver cancer in 1990, he started taking a dose of 450 milligrams of silymarin, or milk thistle, daily, prescribed by his local physician. He had downed it religiously, he said, every day for eleven months. His doctors know of no other successes in treating liver cancer with milk thistle and could find none in the medical literature. Could it be more than coincidence? Did the milk thistle help cure the cancer? Nobody knows. But the doctors agreed that trying milk thistle is reasonable in cases of incurable liver cancer, since it cannot be harmful. And the herb is known to neutralize free radicals and regenerate liver cells.

Unfortunately the carpenter who seemed to have cured his own liver cancer nevertheless died in 1991 of medical complications from an unrelated primary stomach cancer. This does not negate milk thistle's possible anticancer role in the liver. One would not expect the herb to fight off all types of cancer, since its primary activity is in the liver.

How Does It Work?

Milk thistle's active components are a complex of antioxidant bioflavonoids known as silymarin. This unique antioxidant complex exerts its curative powers by both preventing damage to healthy liver cells and stimulating a regeneration of injured liver cells, according to extensive research. Specifically, silymarin stands guard on outer receptor sites of cells, barring toxins from breaking through fatty cell membranes and entering cell interiors. It also neutralizes toxic substances that manage to penetrate cells.

Moreover, it has a unique ability to stimulate protein synthesis in liver cells by increasing genetic (DNA and

RNA) activity. This actually helps regenerate damaged cells. Additionally, milk thistle revs up other antioxidant defenses in liver cells to neutralize toxic invaders. For example, one of the most powerful antioxidants in the body and a major detoxifying substance in the liver is glutathione. In healthy humans silymarin has boosted glutathione concentrations in the liver by 35 percent. Milk thistle also spurs activity of another potent antioxidant, superoxide dismutase, in cells of people with liver disease. Interestingly, this antioxidant appears to be particularly geared to scavenging the type of damaging free radical chemicals that are generated by alcohol in the liver.

A MIRACLE MUSHROOM EXPERIMENT

One way scientists know milk thistle works for sure is that it has saved many people from extinction by the deadly amanita mushroom, also called the death cap. In 1981 German researcher Dr. G. Vogel of the University of Munich conducted a study of forty-nine patients throughout Europe—from Germany, Austria, Italy, Switzerland, and France—who had been poisoned by the mushroom; they were all given injections of milk thistle's active chemicals daily in addition to their regular treatments. Dr. Vogel rightly praised the results as ranging from "amazing to spectacular." Ordinarily the death rate from the poisonous mushroom is 30 to 40 percent. Milk thistle reduced the death rate to zero. Not a single patient died, although victims were usually treated two or three days after the poisoning. This, he said, shows that milk thistle interfered with the circulation of the poison in the liver cells, protecting them from further damage and healing those already damaged.

How Much Do You Need?

Milk thistle extract usually comes as a pill and occasionally as a syrup. The standardized milk thistle extract widely tested in Europe and approved in Germany for liver disease and functional liver impairment contains 70 to 80 percent silymarin. The general recommended dose is 420 milligrams of silymarin taken in three divided doses every day. After you see improvement, as determined by liver function blood tests, you can cut back to a daily dose of 280 milligrams of silymarin. The lower 280 milligrams is also the amount some doctors suggest to help prevent liver dysfunction and damage.

How Quickly Does It Work?

High-quality milk thistle is rapidly absorbed and reaches maximum concentration in the blood about an hour after it is taken. Amazingly, improvement is often noticeable in five to eight days, with a reduction in enzymes and liver size and a lessening of jaundice, yellowing of the skin. A significant reversal of alcoholic liver damage may take a month or two, studies suggest. Essential in judging recovery are blood tests measuring liver enzyme levels, and liver biopsy. Milk thistle depresses elevated liver enzymes, indicating liver cells are healing. Alcoholic patients generally must continue to take milk thistle extract for several months. Remission of chronic persistent hepatitis has been achieved in six months to a year with milk thistle.

The Safety Factor

Unlike other drugs that affect the liver, milk thistle

causes only mild side effects, such as stomach upset, in less than 1 percent of users, according to studies. Most noted is its mild laxative effect, especially in the first few days of use. There is no evidence that milk thistle is toxic or interacts with other medications. Animal studies find no short-term or long-term toxicity at very high doses, including no adverse impact on reproduction, or mutagenic (pro-cancer) activity. Surprisingly, milk thistle is considered so safe in Germany that there are no government warnings against using it, even during pregnancy and lactation.

Consumer Concerns

One good example of standardized milk thistle is Thisilyn from Nature's Way, which contains 70 percent silymarin. It is made by Madaus, a large German company, and has been used in much European research.

Should You Try It?

It makes sense if you have concerns about potential liver damage—if you drink more alcohol than you should, if you have or have had hepatitis or cirrhosis, if you work around industrial chemicals, if you live in an especially polluted environment, and if you are taking pharmaceutical drugs that can cause liver damage, in particular certain cholesterol-lowering drugs, such as Mevacor and Zocor, and certain antidepressants. Indeed, any drug that lists potential liver damage as a side effect might be partly offset by milk thistle extract. If it can strengthen your liver's resistance to such perils of modern civilization, it is well worth trying. If you are at high risk of liver toxicity, a reasonable preventive dose is 280 milligrams of silymarin a day. A therapeutic dose is 420 milligrams daily until the problem is resolved, as determined by medical tests.

Caution: If you have been diagnosed with liver disease, such as hepatitis or cirrhosis, or suspect you may have it, use milk thistle with the supervision of a doctor who can order liver function tests to document that you are improving. Also, it's imperative to curb alcohol intake if you have liver disease or damage.

Mysterious Hay Fever Medicine

(BEE POLLEN)

Nobody knows why it works or how it works, but if it works for you, you can say goodbye to your hay fever—probably forever.

When hay fever season arrives, about one in five Americans would do just about anything to stop the itching, watery eyes, sniffling, and runny nose. Antihistamines and allergy shots are the best orthodox medicine has to offer. But another remedy has attracted a big following among some Americans, including some legislators, purely on the grounds that it seems to work for them, despite any real scientifically controlled studies proving it does. That lack of evidence makes the medical establishment unwilling to endorse it, but to many suffering Americans, including physicians, taking bee pollen or other natural remedies is worth a try, especially if it's the only thing that brings relief.

SENATOR HARKIN'S MIRACLE
An End to Hay Fever Misery

For years Senator Tom Harkin, Democrat of Iowa, tried to conquer his hay fever by taking a prescription antihistamine. Still his allergies grew progressively worse, and the drug stopped working, so his doctor prescribed a stronger dose. But after a year it failed, too. That's why, in the spring of 1993, with the arrival in Washington, D.C., of the cherry blossoms and the high pollen season, the senator was a mess, even though he was gulping down over-the-counter cold and allergy capsules. He had puffy eyes, suffered middle-of-the-night sneezing fits, interrupted public meetings with sniffling, and felt unable to breathe through his clogged nose; he was using half a box of tissues a day.

"I was waking up in the middle of the night. I was sneezing, couldn't breathe. I was using nasal sprays. I was taking Seldane, and it didn't work anymore. I was taking Sudafed and Benadryl. I was driving my wife Ruth nuts," he told the *Des Moines Register*. He was also driving his then-colleague Representative Berkley Bedell of Iowa to distraction with his sneezing. Bedell suggested that Harkin try a remedy, a bee pollen–herb tablet, called Aller-Be-Gone, made by a friend's company. "I was skeptical, but what the heck," said Harkin, "I was tired of taking medicine that didn't work."

He started, per instructions, by downing a few of the bee pollen pills and waiting for ten minutes. (It's imperative to be cautious and go slowly at first to be sure you don't have an allergic reaction to the pollen. See page 149 for safety advice.) Since Senator Harkin didn't get relief, he took a dozen more bee pollen pills. The idea was to repeat the take-and-wait routine until symptoms starting clearing. After downing sixty pills one day, he thought his eyes were itching less. Then, on the sixth day, it happened; his allergy symptoms suddenly stopped cold. To his amazement, his hay fever disappeared. "My nose doesn't run. My eyes are cleared up. I don't sneeze any longer. And I don't take any drugs anymore," he says.

He has continued to pop about six bee pollen pills a day as a preventive, upping the dose at the start of spring and fall pollen seasons, as needed. Although some doctors have told him the bee pollen therapy is nonsense, he refuses to deny his own instant, miraculous cure, bringing incredible relief after years of torment, even if he can't explain it. He admits he doesn't know how the bee pollen product works, but he insists, "I know it cured my allergies. It's a miracle. It's the best thing I've ever seen." On that point, he is firm, sticking with what happened to him, regardless of the lack of mainstream scientific explanation. Senator Harkin's experience bears more weight than that of most others on governmental medical matters. A believer in "alternative" therapies, Harkin was a strong force in establishing NIH's Office of Alternative Medicine to fund and coordinate research into alternative therapies, including bee pollen.

What's the Evidence?

No rigorous scientific studies of the type that convince doctors to use bee pollen for allergies have been done. But several reports in medical journals dating back to 1916 claim that taking bee pollen reduced symptoms of allergies and hay fever. In the 1920s the bee pollen treatment became popular, and one doctor reported he had successfully used it to treat more than 150 cases of asthma and hay fever. In a more recent study, done in 1991 and unpublished, Maurice M. Tinterow, M.D., then with Bio-Communications Research Institute in Wichita, Kansas, and now deceased, tested a pollen product (Bee All Free tablets) on 195 subjects who exhibited symptoms of allergies, asthma, hay fever, chronic sinus condition, and chronic obstructive lung disease. Each subject was given a stopwatch and told to take as many bee pollen tablets as needed until the symptoms disappeared. The bee pollen worked in all but four subjects, said Dr. Tinterow. The average time for the benefit was ten minutes, and the average number of tablets needed was fifteen. One person downed 120 tablets. The quickest effect came for a four-year-old girl; she drank three tablespoons of liquid Bee All Free, in lieu of tablets, and had complete relief in ninety-two seconds. Three subjects—all who got no relief—were mildly nauseated after taking the pills. Dr. Tinterow concluded that the bee pollen effected a permanent cure in most subjects; that is, the symptoms did not return. In those who did have future attacks, he said, taking a little more bee pollen eliminated them.

How Does It Work?

Bee pollen is said to desensitize a person to allergies, much the same way allergy shots do. When your body is exposed to a bit of the offending agent, (allergen or antigen), it marshals immunological defenses or antibiodies against the agent, thus defusing the body's wheezing and sniffling reactions to the allergen. But what particular ingredients (probably proteins) in bee pollen might do the trick are unknown. Dr. Tinterow speculated that it is a combination of many. Nor is the mechanism well studied or defined. But Dr. Tinterow said that in the short run bee pollen produces a "break in the histamine chain," causing the allergy symptoms to disappear instantly. The symptoms do not later reappear, he wrote, because the bee pollen tends to "alter the immune system deficiency" causing the allergy.

DR. JIM GORDON'S MIRACLE
"Honeycomb Cured My Lifelong Allergies"

Dr. James S. Gordon, a Harvard-trained physician and clinical professor in psychiatry and family medicine at the Georgetown University School of Medicine, had suffered "seriously annoying" allergies since he was a kid. They worsened when in the early 1970s he moved to a farm in the vicinity of Washington, D.C. "I was working in the garden and outdoors and there were all kinds of pollens all over the place. I was always taking antihistamines and decongestants, but they never made the allergies any better. They would just relieve symptoms for a while and jazz me up or slow me down." Then he met an Indian healer in London who suggested a remedy recommended in old natural medicine books—honeycomb. Gordon decided to try it as an experiment. "I knew it wasn't going to do me any harm, that's for sure, and—well, as it turned out it did me a lot of good."

He has not had a serious attack of hay fever or pollen allergies for twenty years. His lifelong allergies just disappeared after a few months. Here's how he did it. He bought honeycomb at a local health food store. ("The best is locally produced, so it has exactly the pollens you are going to be sensitive to," he says.) He pressed most of the honey out of the comb, so he wouldn't have to eat "huge doses of honey." He cut the honeycomb roughly into cubic-inch squares and chewed one cube three times a day for three months. "Once you get over the slightly unpleasant waxiness of honeycomb, it's like chewing a different kind of gum," he says.

By the end of the first month he noticed his allergies were lessening. After three months they were virtually gone. And he has not had a serious allergy attack during the twenty-some years since then. If he travels to a place where there are unfamiliar pollens, he may have some reactivity, but not at home around local pollens. "I am minimally affected, if at all," he says. In other words, unlike allergy shots and symptom-relieving pills that must be used regularly for a lifetime, the very short-term use of honeycomb rapidly cured his pollen allergies, presumably forever, by permanently modifying his body's immune responses.

Definitely, it worked better than drugstore antiallergy medicines or allergy shots, he says. But why? "I don't have a clue as to why this works so much better, because we don't know all the things in honeycomb; there's bee pollen, and there may be a dozen other ingredients in there that would not be in allergy shots or bee pollen tablets." Theoretically, he says, the honeycomb is similar to allergy shots, "except it's not shots; it's very natural, precisely designed by nature to work for you. Probably taking a tiny dose this way enables my immune system to mobilize itself, accommodate itself to these allergens, and become immune to them. It's a natural way of establishing immunity."

When asked about any scientifically controlled studies to back up the use of honeycomb to get rid of allergies, Dr. Gordon says frankly that he doesn't know of any, because there is no economic incentive for anyone in the bee and honey industry to spend money to do them. "I didn't try the remedy because there are good controlled studies on it. I did it because it's something herbalists and natural healers have used for centuries. If it works and is harmless [see the next section, about safety], in my view, you don't need double-blind controlled studies to tell you so. I think people should experiment with it themselves and see if it works. It might cure their allergies as it did mine."

The Safety Factor

Some people are allergic to bee stings, which can cause potentially fatal anaphylactic shock. And there are reports of serious allergic reactions to bee pollen. Dr. Daniel Tucker, a board-certified allergist and immunologist in West Palm Beach, Florida, who takes bee pollen himself as a nutritional supplement, agrees there could be a serious risk, including anaphylactic shock, if a person was "sufficiently allergic to one of the pollens or bee antigens." He offers this advice to people who decide to take bee pollen: At first take only a little bit and see if you have any type of allergic reaction. If so, stop taking it. He notes that this is what doctors do when testing for allergies. "We put tiny bits on the skin to see if we get a tiny reaction." If a person is allergic to a substance, the higher the dose, the greater the risk of a bad reaction. That's why you start small and build up. Dr. Tucker also says some people have gastrointestinal upset after taking bee pollen.

Caution: Always start out with very small doses of bee pollen or honeycomb and increase them gradually. If you notice any reactions at all, including skin flushing, headache, or wheezing, stop taking it immediately. If you have had any previous bad reactions to bee stings or bee products, don't try bee pollen, or take it only in the presence of a health professional, advises Dr. Tucker.

Does Dr. Tucker think bee pollen and honeycomb could work? "Sure. It's quite possible that by 'swamping their systems' with antigens in bee pollen, people are desensitizing themselves to some of the agents that trigger hay fever," he says.

Nature's Antinausea Drug

(GINGER)

No question about it, when nausea is a problem, ginger is the best remedy you can find anywhere.

If you tend to have motion sickness on boats, planes, cars, or elsewhere, or suffer from nausea occasionally, your first choice of a miracle cure should be ginger. Ginger is the safest, oldest, and most effective antinausea remedy known. It appears to work primarily on the digestive system, not the brain, and thus lacks the bothersome nervous system side effects, such as drowsiness, that you typically get from over-the-counter drugs. That ginger fights nausea of all kinds is evident from centuries of usage, controlled scientific studies, and raves from people who have tried it.

JUDY'S MIRACLE
"I'm Not Afraid of Getting Sick Anymore"

Although she had taken short domestic flights before, Judy Stevens, then age thirty, knew she was in trouble when she made her first transatlantic flight with her husband on a vacation from Baltimore to London about twenty years ago. Soon after takeoff, her stomach became extremely queasy, and she was nauseated for most of the eight-hour trip. She dreaded thinking of the return trip. Motion sickness in the air and on the water was a part of her life. "On planes, even big ones, I get nauseated, I feel like I want to vomit." A couple of years later on a Mexican vacation, she went deep-sea fishing, took a Dramamine to keep down the nausea, and became so drowsy she slept on the deck all day, missing the entire experience.

Since she did not fly regularly, motion sickness was not a constant concern. Then in the 1990s she began making more frequent hops on a small commuter plane from Hagerstown, Maryland, to make connections in Baltimore to fly south to visit relatives. "That was worse. On a small plane, I get really anxious and sick because it bounces around more." Then someone told her about ginger. The first time she tried it, she simply dissolved about half a teaspoon of ground ginger in tea before takeoff and carried extra ginger to put in tea at airports where she had to change planes. She was amazed. "It really worked. I had absolutely no queasiness, no anxiety, no nausea, nothing. When I take ginger I'm just fine."

On one trip in the spring of 1994 she took her thirteen-year-old granddaughter, Jessica, with her, stopping in two airports before the final destination. Jessica had a history of motion sickness in cars. To make taking the ginger easier, Judy bought 500-milligram ginger capsules. They each took two capsules twenty to thirty minutes before boarding the plane. "Jessica had no signs of motion sickness. It was the most pleasant trip for both of us," says Judy. "I'll tell you, it's just remarkable. I don't know what I would do without ginger. There was only once, in extreme turbulence on a commuter flight, when I got sick, but everybody else was worse off. I don't think anything would have helped in that case. But the rest of the time I can't say enough for ginger; it works 100 percent for me. I feel great now when I get on the plane and when I get off the plane."

FRED'S MIRACLE
"Ginger Saved Me When Drugs Did Not"

For fourteen years Fred Thomas, age thirty-three, had been in agony; the NSAIDS (nonsteroidal anti-inflammatory drugs) he took to relieve the pain of his rheumatoid disorder made him so nauseated he was unable to eat anything until about seven at night. He also had severe diarrhea. "It's a constant feeling—the feeling of being sick," says Thomas, a full-time computer science student in Portsmouth, England. Unfortunately, the drug Indocin that best relieved the pain in his hips and spine from his disease, known as ankylosing spondylitis, also produced the worst upset stomach. He tried several drugs to combat the upset stomach, but none worked. "I tried everything, all the tablets my local GP prescribed."

Then one day in late 1993 he noticed ginger capsules in a cupboard, left over from the time his wife, Allison, took them for morning sickness. "Perhaps it's worth giving it a go," he said to himself. So he took one capsule.

"You would not believe how different I felt after

just one pill. It was absolutely incredible. I felt really good, almost as if I'd gone back to before I had all this trouble with my stomach." He was able to get up in the morning and eat for the first time in three years. He still takes a ginger capsule when he gets up and one when he goes to bed. Although the ginger has not entirely cured his nausea, it has made a dramatic difference. "Nothing else, no other drugs, compared to what the ginger did for me. I can't push it strongly enough. Anyone who is feeling any type of problem with the stomach should try it. And it's cheap. It costs me about 10 pence a capsule [about 15 cents]. Also, I've experienced no side effects from the ginger at all.

"I had heard before of letting children eat ginger biscuits [cookies] on car trips to settle their stomach, but I thought it was just an old wives' tale. It's definitely not. I would recommend ginger to anybody with stomach problems."

What Is It?

Gingerroot, or, more accurately, the rhizome (underground stem) of the ginger plant, has been used in China, India, and other Asian countries for twenty-five centuries to aid digestion and relieve nausea, and is widely accepted as an antinausea medication by health authorities and practitioners in many other countries.

Ginger is approved by Germany's governmental Commission E for antimotion sickness and indigestion; about 400,000 capsules of ginger are sold annually in that country to combat motion sickness. In Denmark about 14 million capsules are sold yearly as a government-endorsed treatment for "rheumatism and travel sickness." Ginger is considered an over-the-counter remedy in the United Kingdom.

What's the Evidence?

Pioneering studies by Utah psychologist Daniel Mowrey, published in the British medical journal *The Lancet* in 1982, established scientific credibility for the antinausea effects of ginger. Mowrey found that subjects put in a tilted rotating chair were less likely to get sick if given about 1,000 milligrams of ginger powder (two capsules) beforehand, rather than Dramamine or a dummy pill (placebo.)

Another test of eighty Danish naval cadets showed that those who took ginger capsules—a scant one-half teaspoon of ground ginger—about half an hour before hitting rough seas staved off seasickness better than those getting a placebo. Ginger suppressed vomiting by 72 percent and overall was about 38 percent protective against seasickness. The protection lasted about four hours.

Nausea resulting from anesthesia after surgery is a problem in about 30 percent of patients. But ginger is a solution there, too, according to research. In a controlled study British physician M. E. Bone at St. Bartholomew's Hospital in London found that ginger (about one-third of a teaspoon) was better at preventing postoperative nausea in a group of sixty women than the often used injections of the tranquilizer metoclopramide. A 1993 study of 120 patients undergoing surgery showed the same thing. Ginger has also been shown effective in suppressing nausea and vomiting associated with chemotherapy, according to a study at the University of Alabama.

FIGHTING MORNING SICKNESS

Some health professionals, including obstetricians, now recommend a little ginger to fight morning sickness—

nausea and vomiting during early pregnancy. The persuasive reasons: It usually works and appears much less likely to be teratogenic (capable of inducing birth defects) than other antinausea drugs used in pregnancy. One controlled German study of 27 women found ginger effective in "hyperemesis gravidarum," a severe form of nausea and vomiting related to pregnancy, in about 70 percent of subjects. Taking 250 milligrams of gingerroot powder in capsules four times a day reduced the severity of nausea and the number of vomiting attacks in cases of early pregnancy (less than twenty weeks). The authors said they found no reason for concern in their studies or others in the medical literature that ginger could harm the fetus. Stephen Fulder, Ph.D., a British expert on herbal medicines, after an exhaustive review of the medical literature in 1996, pronounced "normal doses" of ginger "completely safe in pregnancy." Nevertheless, pregnant women should always consult a doctor before taking any medicinal agent, including ginger.

How Does It Work?

No one is sure what constituents in ginger are responsible for its antinausea effect. But two compounds—shogaols and gingerols—isolated from gingerroot have had antiemetic (antinausea) properties in animals. General scientific opinion holds that ginger works almost entirely in the digestive tract, although it may have a slight depressant effect on the central nervous system, according to a recent study of frogs.

How Much Do You Need?

To prevent nausea and vomiting from motion sickness, take two 500-milligram ginger capsules about half an hour before boarding a plane, a boat, or another vehicle.

Take another one or two if you become nauseated later. The initial dose should ward off symptoms for about four hours.

The Safety Factor

Ginger has been safely used for centuries as a food and medication. No human studies have reported any adverse effects from ginger, nor are there any cases of ginger toxicity on record in the medical literature. In animal studies, ginger is not toxic even at very high doses. Thus ginger is listed as GRAS (generally recognized as safe) by the FDA. However, research shows that ginger has anticoagulant activity, thinning the blood. Thus people with bleeding problems or on anticoagulants should exercise caution in taking high amounts of ginger. Excessive ginger may also raise blood pressure and be detrimental to those with gallstones, say German authorities.

Caution: If you are pregnant, use ginger for morning sickness only on the advice of a doctor, and don't consume more than 1,000 milligrams daily, the dose used safely in studies. Using ginger to counteract nausea during chemotherapy to treat cancer could promote gastrointestinal bleeding when platelet count is low. Always check with a doctor before using ginger during chemotherapy.

What's the Alternative?

All antinausea ingredients in over-the counter drugs currently approved by the FDA act on the central nervous system and thus carry side effects, including dizziness, tinnitus, lassitude (weariness), incoordination, fatigue, blurred vision, euphoria, nervousness, insomnia, and tremors. Further, you should not use these drugs if you have asthma, emphysema, or other respiratory problems.

Nor should you combine them with alcohol, sedatives, or tranquilizers. Ginger has none of these drawbacks. "Unlike other antinausea medications that act centrally, ginger appears to act directly on the digestive system, and therefore has none of the troubling central nervous system side effects found with conventional antiemetic drugs," points out a recent petition by the European-American Phytomedicines Coalition to have ginger approved as an over-the-counter drug.

Consumer Concerns
On the basis of recent scientific evidence and longtime safe effective usage in other countries, the European-American Phytomedicines Coalition in 1995 petitioned the U.S. Food and Drug Administration to designate ginger an over-the-counter remedy for nausea and motion sickness. By 1997, despite compelling scientific evidence, the FDA had not approved it.

What Else Is It Good For?
Ginger has versatile pharmacological activity. It acts as an anticoagulant and anti-inflammatory agent. Investigations by Dr. Krishna C. Srivastava of Odense University in Denmark have found that both fresh gingerroot and the ground spice (less than a teaspoon a day) can relieve arthritis symptoms and help prevent migraine headaches, probably because of its anti-inflammatory activity.

Exotic New Tranquilizer

(K A V A)

**This magic pill from the South Seas is a new way
to deal with stress and anxiety.**

Tense? Anxious? Need help calming down and relaxing—or falling into a deep, sound sleep? Stress is a
constant companion in modern life. In an instant our
adrenal glands can send a burst of adrenaline and other
hormones to pump up our bodies to handle a perceived
danger (it's a primitive survival mechanism called the
fight-or-flight response). But the flood of chemicals that
causes our hearts to pound and our blood pressure to rise
is usually overkill for the mundane reality of the situation:
everyday frustration on the superhighway, anxiety over a
work deadline, worry about overdue bills, the screaming
siren of a police car. Some of us live in a state of chronic
stress or have anxiety disorder, even panic attacks, and are
in a frantic search for relief. The solution is sometimes
alcohol, painkillers, prescription antianxiety drugs, tranquilizers such as Xanax and Valium, and sleeping pills,
such as Halcion.

They all bring relief at a potentially high price: addiction, confusion, loss of concentration and memory, and
withdrawal symptoms.

But you may also find help in a highly unusual herbal remedy, used for centuries in the South Pacific and now widely tested in Europe. It is an increasingly popular herbal alternative to high-octane pharmaceutical agents. An exotic herb called kava may soothe your nerves and relieve anxiety just as well as prescription tranquilizers without the same risky side effects and high cost. Kava, many users say, induces mild euphoria, reduces agitation, takes away aches by relaxing muscles in the back, neck, and jaw, and brings on a wonderful, refreshing sleep.

MARK'S MIRACLE
"It's Great for No-Stress Sleep"

Mark Blumenthal is as energetic as they come, always fast-talking, funny, exuberant, exploding to communicate his passion for herbs and his mission to have them elevated to their rightful place in America's health system. As head of the American Botanical Council in Austin, Texas, Blumenthal jets around the world, attending meeting after meeting on the pharmacology and politics of herbs. And he loses a lot of sleep. To make up for it, he has for years taken kava to produce a "deep restful sleep" when he knows he will not be able to get his normal quota of snoozes.

"When I go to bed late, knowing I have to be up early after only a few hours of sleep, I usually take two or three squirts of a liquid kava tincture before retiring. For example, yesterday I flew from Austin to Boston. The plane was late taking off; we sat on the tarmac for three hours for repairs. By the time I got to my hotel in Boston, it was almost three A.M., and I had to be at a meeting by eight A.M. I took kava before I went to bed, knowing I would wake up fully rested and refreshed after just four hours or so of sleep, because it helps you get that critical REM sleep. Kava reduces anxiety; it's a nice muscle relaxant, but the great thing is that your head still stays very clear. It's wonderful stuff!"

There is no other plant like kava that gives such utter relaxation while at the same time allowing such clear penetrating mindfulness."—Oregon herbal authority Peggy Brevoort

What Is It?

Kava is the root of a shrub belonging to the same plant family as black pepper. It's native to the South Pacific islands and has been used there for centuries as a ceremonial and celebratory nonalcoholic calming drink to bring on relaxation and sociability. Medicinally it's been used in the South Pacific to treat gonorrhea, bronchitis, and rheumatism. In Europe it's widely used as a mild sedative—a safer substitute for prescription benzodiazepine tranquilizers and sleeping pills, such as Valium, Xanax, Halcion, Librium, and Dalmane—to treat anxiety, mental stress, and insomnia.

Medicinal plant expert Kerry Bone, technical director and a founder of MediHerb, Australia's largest producer of botanical medicines, recently described kava's effects in an article in the *British Journal of Phytotherapy*. In small doses, he says, kava creates a mild euphoria, relaxation, and restful sleep. "The kava beverage first causes a numbing and astringent effect in the mouth," wrote Bone. "This is followed by a relaxed, sociable state where fatigue and anxiety are lessened. Eventually a deep restful sleep ensues from which the user awakens the next morning refreshed and without a hangover." However, Bone also notes, "Excessive consumption can lead to dizziness and stupefaction, and a syndrome of kava abuse has been described."

What Is It Good For?

Kava in proper doses is best at relieving anxiety; most important, it works without robbing you of alertness. It also gets high marks as a safe plant relaxant of skeletal muscle, and thus is good for treating muscle spasms and tension headaches. It alleviates mild insomnia because it's an excellent hypnotic. Kava is approved in Germany as an over-the-counter drug for "conditions of nervous anxiety, stress, and restlessness." The United Kingdom lists kava on the General Sales List of approved herbal medicines.

What's the Evidence?

Fifty years of research—dozens of excellent studies, most done in Germany—show unquestionably that kava is a psychoactive substance—a mood elevator and mild sedative. Starting in the late 1950s experiments proved that kava extracts, and its principal chemicals, put animals to sleep and produced brain waves in humans similar to those induced by antianxiety drugs. However, unlike Valium-type tranquilizers, kava mysteriously induces sleep without causing sedation. One theory is that kava affects different receptor sites in the brain than Valium-type drugs do. Tests also show that kava relaxes both skeletal and smooth muscles.

Undeniably, kava works in humans, according to many well-controlled so-called double-blind placebo studies, the gold standard of science. For example, such a well-conducted 1996 trial of fifty-eight German patients with anxiety (not caused by psychotic disorders) found that a dose of 100 milligrams of kava extract (standardized to 70 milligrams of kavalactones) three times a day significantly relieved anxiety. Subjects were dramatically better after only one week of kava therapy, and improved increasingly during the four-week study. In another recent test of eighty-four anxiety sufferers, 400 milligrams a day of a kava product, known as Kavain, improved memory and reaction time. Kava was also effective in reducing anxiety, depression, and other symptoms among forty menopausal German women in a 1991 study.

How does it compare with conventional drugs? Kava is as effective as prescription tranquilizers, according to comparative controlled double-blind tests. In one instance thirty-eight patients with anxiety due to neurotic disturbances took either kava as Kavain or oxazepam, a benzodiazepine tranquilizer of the Valium family. Kava equaled the tranquilizer in reducing anxiety according to established measures of its antianxiety action. Both agents caused patients to improve progressively in anxiety scores over a four-week period.

Further, kava proves superior to Valium-like tranquilizers because kava does not dope you up, robbing you of mental alertness, research shows. A 1993 double-blind test by German scientist H. J. Heinze, a leading researcher on kava, indeed found that after taking the prescription tranquilizer oxazepam, subjects had slower and less accurate responses on psychometric tests. This was not true after they took kava. Just the opposite: Kava improved their reaction times and performance on memory tests. And there's much less worry about becoming drowsy after taking kava than after taking tranquilizers. Forty healthy people who took standardized extract of kava showed no dimunition in their ability to drive or operate machines.

Nor did a standardized dose of kava aggravate the effects of a little alcohol, as do tranquilizers.

A 1994 study of twelve volunteers by German investigators compared kava extract (standardized on 120 milligrams of kava pyrones) with 10 milligrams of Valium. Both produced similar increases in slow brain waves, according to electroencephalogram (EEG) mappings of the brain, and a decrease of intensity of alpha waves. Valium worked faster, producing maximum brain effects after two hours. Kava's effects peaked at six hours. However, only kava improved subjects' scores on simple reaction-time tests and complex multiple-choice reaction tests, indicating once again that kava calms without sedating and ruining mental acuity.

How Does It Work?

Psychoactive chemicals in kava are fairly well identified; they are specific chemicals called kavalactones. In tests on animals and humans they produce sedative, hypnotic, and anticonvulsant effects on the brain, as measured by EEGs. However, the agents don't act in the same fashion on brain cells or in the same area of the brain as human-made tranquilizers and antidepressants do. An important German EEG study of brain waves suggested that kava appears to work at the deepest level of the brain on the limbic structures, known to regulate emotions. This may help explain why kava is considered a mood elevator.

How Much Do You Need?

Be sure to get kava products that are standardized to contain a certain amount of the active kavalactones. This will be noted on the label. At times of stressful events or to relieve anxiety, a daily dose equal to 180 milligrams of kavalactones should be sufficient, say experts. If a pill contains 60 milligrams of kavalactones, that would mean one pill three times a day. That is the amount used in most studies as a general tranquilizer or antianxiety agent. You generally notice a relaxing effect rather quickly—within half an hour or so, say experts. To bring on sleep, a single dose of the 120 to 180 kavalactones taken an hour before going to bed is usually enough, says kava expert Kerry Bone. "If I have jet lag and can't go to sleep, I take two or three tablets of standardized extract and find it very effective," he says.

The Safety Factor

In general therapeutic doses, Germany's health officials declare kava free of known adverse side effects, except a yellow discoloration of skin, hair, and nails if you take it continuously for too long. The yellow disappears when you stop using the herb. Also possible, but rare: allergic skin reactions, enlargement of pupils, and disturbances of physical equilibrium. German health officials recommend against taking kava continuously for more than three months without a doctor's advice. Also, high doses taken for a long time can cause a peculiar skin condition in which the skin becomes dry and scaly, especially on the palms, soles, forearms, and back.

Don't take kava if you are pregnant, nursing (obviously, it could be passed on to a baby through mother's milk), or suffering from endogenous depression, or if you have Parkinson's disease. Further, herbal authority Dr. Donald Brown of Seattle advises against taking kava in combination with any substances that have an effect on the central nervous system; this includes alcohol, prescription drugs, such as tranquilizers and antidepressants, and botanical medicines, such as St. John's wort and Valerian.

Special caution: Although kava is not addictive as alcohol, illicit drugs, and some pharmaceuticals are, the possibility of kava abuse is real. In excessive doses kava can cause signs of drunkenness. Recently a man was arrested in Salt Lake City for driving under the influence of kava. He had allegedly become intoxicated after drinking sixteen cups of kava tea. Australian kava authority Kerry Bone says kava abuse syndrome is increasing in many South Sea islands, such as Fiji, and in certain populations in Australia. Such abusers are taking three to five times the therapeutic dose, or around fifteen standard pills a day, he says.

What Else Is It Good For?
Experiments suggest that kava is a strong analgesic—that is, it may help control pain—although clinical studies have not been done. Some people use it to treat stress-related muscle pain, such as backache, neck ache, and TMJ, a painful condition of the jaw and head.

The Antabuse of Plants

(K U D Z U)

It makes Chinese alcohol abusers and laboratory animals go on the wagon. It might do the same for you. Scientific tests on humans are just getting under way.

Surely any agent—from prescription drug to over-the-counter herbal remedy—would be a welcome cure for our epidemic of alcoholism, which inflicts immeasurable human misery and, often death. Despite much looking, no such nostrums have emerged. Most drug treatments including antidepressants and Antabuse have largely failed and carry the risk of side effects. But now scientists at top medical centers, at Harvard and the University of North Carolina, believe they have found a promising new pharmacological treatment for alcohol abuse—one used in China for more than 1,300 years—the kudzu plant.

What Is It?
Kudzu is a tenacious traveling vine of the legume family that spreads so quickly, especially in warm climates, including the southern part of the United States, that poet James Dickey called it "a vegetable form of cancer." Its starchy root tubers have been used as a medication in

China since 200 B.C. It has a special reputation for combating drunkenness, as noted in the Chinese Pharmacopeia of A.D. 600.

What's the Evidence?
Tests on humans are just getting under way in the United States, but kudzu definitely discourages drinking in laboratory animals, and has long been used in China as a cure for drunkenness. Even today kudzu is a common treatment for alcoholism in China, and many Chinese patients and traditional physicians, also called herbalists, rave about its effectiveness. But since such practitioners do not keep records on patients or publish their findings, it's tough to amass scientific evidence to validate its value, says Dr. Wing-Ming Keung, a biochemist at Harvard Medical School. He decided to search out the evidence himself.

On a recent investigative trip to his native Hong Kong, Dr. Keung interviewed thirteen modern and traditional physicians or herbalists and compiled 300 cases of patients with chronic alcoholism who had been treated with kudzu tea or kudzu-based medications. "In all cases," Dr. Keung reported, "the medications were considered effective in both controlling and suppressing appetite for alcohol and improving the function of alcohol-affected vital organs. No toxic side effects were reported by the Chinese physicians." Actually, the kudzu significantly reduced the craving for alcohol in a week, he reported. Even more impressively, after two to four weeks 80 percent of the alcoholics said their craving for alcohol was completely gone.

This inspired Dr. Keung and Harvard professor Bert L. Vallee to perform the first scientific test of kudzu on a strain of hamsters known to have an innate fondness for alcohol. Offered water or alcohol, these animals down the booze every time in huge amounts—comparable to a human's drinking five cases of wine a day. But, as the researchers reported in 1993, when the animals were first given kudzu extract and then exposed to the alcohol, they drank only half as much! Moreover, the alcoholic animals had the same aversion to alcohol after they were primed with two compounds, daidzin and daidzein, extracted from kudzu root. When they no longer got their daily kudzu, they went back to their boozy habits. "We thought this was rather dramatic," said Dr. Vallee.

A TEA TO SOBER YOU UP?

In 1996 a team of investigators at the University of North Carolina at Chapel Hill and Research Triangle Park also found that kudzu worked in their lab animals. When alcohol-loving rats were given kudzu either orally or by injection, they, too, drank about half as much as usual. The scientists also noted that kudzu suppressed alcohol's intoxicating effects after it entered the bloodstream, tending to confirm the ancient claim that taking kudzu before imbibing alcohol helps stave off intoxication and hangovers. In fact, the idea for the study was triggered by Dr. David Lee, a natural products chemist at Chapel Hill's Research Triangle Institute, after he visited China and noted that kudzu is included in a "morning after tea," known as xing-jiu-ling, which essentially means "sober up." The investigators used imported Chinese kudzu processed to extract what they believe are the primary active agents.

More exciting, the North Carolina research team, directed by Dr. Amir Rezvani, associate professor of psychiatry at the university, then tested kudzu in monkeys, our closest biological cousins; the herb depressed their desire for alcohol, too. After hooking test monkeys on alcohol, researchers gave them the kudzu for a week. On kudzu the monkeys reduced their intake of alcohol about 25 percent, according to Dr. Lee. That's as good as or better than the drug naltrexone does, he claims. (Naltrexone is also approved by the FDA to treat alcoholism.) Since monkeys are biologically almost identical to humans, researchers take it for granted that what works in primates works in humans. That's what makes the new monkey findings so compelling. Still, the researchers' next step is a controlled scientific test of kudzu on human alcoholics. Such studies are needed to convince the general community and to determine the proper dosage for humans, says Dr. Lee. "We must figure out how much of the kudzu compounds humans need to get a benefit."

What makes kudzu especially appealing is its lack of side effects. Naltrexone can cause liver damage. And Antabuse works precisely through its side effect of creating nausea and vomiting. "That's the best part of this kudzu," says Dr. Lee, "It's so safe. There's no liver toxicity."

"As often happens with remedies of this kind that have been used by the populace for millennia, this one had been ignored by modern science," said Harvard's Dr. Vallee. "It's good to look at nature and folk medicine and realize nature has lots to teach us," agrees Dr. Hans Jornvall, a leading alcohol researcher at Sweden's Karolinska Institute in Stockholm.

How Does It Work?
Western efforts to dissect the active components in kudzu have had puzzling results. The Harvard researchers declared two similar compounds—daidzein and mainly daidzin—in kudzu responsible for its ability to curtail alcohol intake in hamsters. Further, they showed that daidzin affects enzymes that metabolize, or break down,

alcohol in the body. Specifically, daidzin blocks an enzyme that breaks down acetaldehyde, a by-product of alcohol taken into the body. That made a lot of sense because a buildup of acetaldehyde in the body is what causes nausea in someone who drinks alcohol and takes disulfiram, better known as Antabuse. Thus it appeared that kudzu worked just like Antabuse, one of two drugs approved in the United States to treat alcohol abuse. However, the Harvard researchers did not detect any accumulation of the nausea-triggering chemical in their guzzling hamsters. Apparently kudzu does not work like Antabuse by creating nausea, which makes it all the more appealing. The Harvard researchers are back to square one in understanding how kudzu works.

On the other hand, the North Carolina researchers are working on a different theory. They have isolated and patented three different active kudzu compounds that they say work in a different fashion, directly on the nervous system, to discourage cravings. Dr. Rezvani theorizes that the kudzu compounds boost natural opiates in the brain, including serotonin and dopamine, lessening alcohol cravings. He points out that people with low levels of these neurotransmitters tend to crave alcohol. If so, kudzu might also help suppress cravings for other addictive substances, including cigarettes, hard drugs, and even certain foods.

The Safety Factor

Kudzu's toxicity is very low. Taking as much as 100 grams, or 3.5 ounces, had no adverse effects, according to one study. Don't combine kudzu with prescription drugs, cautions Dr. Keung, unless your physician okays it. The herb can alter the way such drugs are metabolized. As with any unusual substance, kudzu should not be consumed by pregnant women unless it is approved by their doctors.

Consumer Concerns

In China kudzu is sold as a root or extract. There, as well as in the United States, you can buy extracts from a health food store. It comes in a rectangular cube, a tincture, and a pill form. Such crude extracts will probably help to avoid hangovers and to discourage alcohol abuse, says Dr. Lee. However, the proper dose is quite unclear. In China tablets are standardized so that 10 milligrams equals 5 grams of crude root. Some experts have advised taking one such standardized tablet two or three times a day to discourage drinking.

Should You Try It?

True, at this writing, there are no scientifically controlled human studies on kudzu. But can the human experience of a whole population of Chinese be totally wrong? The centuries of use in China, now coupled with convincing new animal evidence that kudzu works, add weight to its probable effectiveness in humans. However, its use is still very much trial and error in treating alcoholism, since there's no sure way to know the best type and dose. There seems little risk in trying it as a remedy for hangover, or to see if it dampens the desire for alcohol. But it is clearly not a substitute for conventional alcoholism treatment, although it might be incorporated as part of a total alcohol treatment program.

What Else Is It Good For?

Kudzu might also be good for the heart. Research shows that kudzu chemicals and root extracts display protective pharmacological activity; they can dilate coronary and cerebral vessels, increasing blood flow and blood oxygen supply. There are reports that the herb has lowered blood pressure in humans and animals. Kudzu also has antioxidant activity that might help retard artery clogging. In China kudzu has been used for centuries to treat headaches, high blood pressure, mild fevers, allergies, diarrhea, angina (chest pain) and stomach upset, although no Western-style studies have been done to support these medicinal uses.

The Universal
Miracle Cure

(FISH OIL OR OMEGA-3S)

**It can fix up your heart, blood, joints, colon, even
your brain. It's a unique and potent medicine.**

Your joints are arthritic and painful. You have colitis or
inflammatory bowel disease. Your heart rhythm is
abnormal, making you vulnerable to sudden death from
heart attack. Your blood triglycerides are too high or your
blood vessels are slightly clogged and you're afraid an
artery may clamp shut, triggering a heart attack or stroke.
Your mood or mental functioning is not great—you're a
little depressed, edgy, and irritable; you don't concentrate
as well as you once did; or you feel unfocused.

You may need one of nature's most marvelous, versatile medicines—those unique fatty molecules found in
fish. Remarkable new research is finding that this peculiar
type of fat is so essential to your cells that they malfunction without it, creating a cascade of events that cripple
you in ways quite unsuspected until lately. It is no exagger-
ation to say that fish oil or its major unique component,
omega-3-fatty acids, is such an extraordinary pharmacological substance that your body collapses without it.

The reason: Fish oil, along with other types of fat in the
membranes encapsulating cells, literally controls the cell's

behavior. And as each cell goes, so goes the rest of the body. A minuscule imbalance of fatty acids in individual cells can make them go berserk, creating chaos throughout your body.

Only in the last decade have scientists begun to understand how the fat content of cells can foster illness and how infusing cells with the right fat can correct the fatty imbalance, making dysfunctional cells behave properly and disease symptoms subside. Among other things, the omega-3 fatty acids in fish temper our cells' angry inflammatory attacks on other cells, keep cell membranes pliable enough to slip easily through blood vessels, rev up antioxidant defenses, and modulate the passage of electro-chemical messages through brain and heart cells.

True, omega-3 fish oil defies the definition of conventional drugs because it does not conform to the pharmaceutical mind-set that one agent treats only a single specific symptom or disorder. Fish oil's therapeutic powers are so broad they might seem preposterous were they not so scientifically grounded. Leading scientists throughout the world acknowledge that fish oil is a therapeutic wizard, full of surprises.

What Is It?

The particular type of fatty acid in fish oil is unique. It is called long-chain omega-3. Some plant foods—rapeseed (canola oil), flaxseed, walnuts—also have omega-3s that are not as potent as those in fish. Additionally, fish oil or omega-3s are of two types—EPA, long touted as crucial in heart disease; and DHA, now known to be important in brain functions. You get these fish oils when you eat fatty fish, such as mackerel, sardines, salmon, and herring. Fish oil, containing specific amounts of omega-3 fatty acids, is also put into soft-gel capsules that you can take therapeutically.

How Does It Work?

Astounding as it may seem, the type of fatty acids in your cells orchestrate a myriad events that determine your well-being. Most critical is the balance of types of fatty acids in cells. Too much of one type of oil, called omega–6 (dominant in corn oil, for example), causes them to spew off inflammatory chemicals that stab pains into your joints and inflame the inner lining of your intestinal tract. Whereas omega-3 oils, dominant in fish, tends to subdue inflammation—a process underlying a broad spectrum of diseases such as arthritis, asthma, colitis, psoriasis, and even artery disease. Fish oil also spurs release of chemicals that can influence electrical activity in the heart as well as soothe the brain, lift the mood, and focus the mind.

NEW BRAIN BREAKTHROUGHS

Although for years scientists understood that fish oil could lighten the burden of heart disease, arthritis and other inflammatory diseases, only recently have they focused on the impact of fish oil in the brain. New evidence shows that fish oil may also be therapeutic for mood and brain disturbances. Dr. Norman Salem at the National Institute of Mental health says low levels of omega-3s, especially one fraction called DHA, which is rich in salmon, are linked to depression, aggressive behavior, brain damage from alcohol, attention deficit disorder, and possibly Alzheimer's disease. Too little DHA and other omega-3 fat in brain cell membranes, says Dr. Salem, may compromise proper brain functioning in various ways. He explains that DHA fatty acid helps regulate cell membrane functions involved in transmitting signals among brain cells. It's easier, research suggests, for brain chemicals such as serotonin to transmit proper messages when the consistency of fat in membranes surrounding brain cells is fluid and flexible, as is fish oil, rather than stiff and hardened like lard.

If you don't feed brain cell membranes enough of the right type of fat, the messages can be short-circuited and garbled. That may mean a disturbance in mood, concentration, memory, attention, and behavior. Such omega-3 fats are also critical to proper brain development in the fetus, infants, and young children and even to brain functions in adults. It appears, as the old adage says, that fish is truly "brain food," says Dr. Salem.

ATTENTION DEFICIT PUZZLE
Youngsters deficient in omega-3 oils are more apt to have behavioral and learning problems or attention deficit and hyperactivity disorder (ADHA), according to recent research at Purdue University. Investigators Laura Stevens and John R. Burgess tested the omega-3 blood levels of ninety-six boys, ages six to twelve; about half had been identified as having ADHD. Clearly, Stevens and Burgess say, "boys with lower levels of the omega-3 fat scored higher in frequency of behavioral problems," including hyperactivity, impulsivity, anxiety, temper tantrums, and sleep problems.

Does taking more omega-3 and other appropriate fats cure the deficiency and improve ADHD behavior? Burgess and Stevens as well as other scientists in Great Britain have studies under way to find out. It seems clear that in some youngsters it does work. Dr. Salem agrees there's scientific reason for trying it. "Fatty acids in brain cells are powerful stuff," he says.

RICHARD'S AND JAY'S
DOUBLE MIRACLE
Up from Academic Failure
to Graduation with Honors

When her two sons, Richard and Jay, were mere toddlers, three years apart, Jennifer Hill* recognized that they were both hyperactive and disruptive and couldn't calm down enough to play with toys and games. By the time the boys were in school, she felt they were headed for academic disaster. Richie was diagnosed with learning disabilities and was put in a special education class. Desperate, his mother tried everything, including the famous Feingold diet that cut out sugar, chocolate, milk, and food additives. It helped, but it was not totally successful.

Reluctantly, she put eight-year-old Richard on the recommended drug Ritalin; he seemed to get worse. The younger Jay was in trouble also—"with severe temper outbursts and speech delay." He went on Ritalin too with little success. Then Richie at age twelve "started developing severe migraine-like headaches."

That's when a doctor friend told the Hills about two pioneering doctors, Sidney Baker and Leo Galland at the Gesell Institute of Human Development in New Haven, Connecticut. "They did all kinds of biochemical tests on Richie," says his mother, "and found that he had a very unusual fatty acid profile. So they put him on large doses of fish oil capsules, up to 12 grams a day, and his headaches started to disappear. He also got flaxseed oil and primrose oil, which made him feel calmer and better generally."

The doctors tested Jay and found him also deficient in fatty acids, in a slightly different way; he too, started taking fish oil capsules, the MaxEpa brand, and flaxseed oil. His mother vivdly remembers how "really well it worked;" the next year Jay's scores on a national achievement test jumped from the 60th percentile to the 90th percentile. "My husband and I were so excited," says Jennifer. It marked the beginning of a new era for the Hill family.

Richard overcame his "learning disability," graduating third in his high school class and later with honors from a major midwestern university. He is working on a doctorate degree. Jay, too, graduated in the top 10 percent of his high school class, and was a Phi Beta Kappa at a prestigious university in California. "It just completely turned their lives around," says their mother. "It's enough to make me cry when I think how differently it could have turned out. It could have been so disastrous if we had not found out about the fatty acid deficiencies and corrected them. It's hard to believe that a little fat can have such a monumental effect on a child's brain and behavior, but it can—we know." Richard and Jay, now in their mid-twenties, still religiously take capsules of fish oil and flaxseed oil in relatively low doses to keep their blood fatty acids in normal balance.

*Note: pseudonyms are used to protect the privacy of the family.

About the case: At the time, fifteen years ago, when these boys' behavior was treated with essential fatty acids, virtually nothing was known about their pharmacological effects on the brain, but thanks to some pioneering doctors, who picked up on early clues in the medical literature, it was an experiment that paid off. And now scientists understand that fatty acids can affect brain cells and possibly modify behavior. Although much research needs to be done on the connection between fatty acid deficiency and the brain and behavior, for other parents with troubled children it is a reasonable possibility to be explored.

IF YOU WANT TO TRY
FATTY ACIDS FOR ADHD
Advice from Purdue researchers
John Burgess and Laura Stevens

- First, try to determine if your child with ADHD has a fatty acid deficiency. The primary signs are: excessive thirst; frequent urination; dry skin; dry unmanageable "strawlike" hair; dandruff; small hard bumps on the arms, thighs, or elbows.
- Increase the amount of essential fatty acids in your child's diet. This includes eating more canola oil, flaxseed oil, and most importantly, more omega-3 fish oil, as found in salmon, fresh tuna, mackerel, and sardines. The precise amount, if any, of which fatty acids might help a child with ADHD is quite unclear at this point and is largely a matter of trial and error. Research is under way to find out.
- Don't take your child off a pharmaceutical drug, such as Ritalin, and substitute fatty acids without first consulting a health professional.
- Don't count on omega-3 and other fatty acids to solve your child's ADHD problems. ADHD is a complex syndrome, and treatment entails other factors, including

behavior modifications. It's also unclear how much of what type oils each individual child may need.

- *Bottom line:* If you want to try fatty acid supplements with an ADHD youngster, work with health professionals and don't stop other treatments or medications without proper medical advice.

AMAZING NEW HEART DISCOVERIES

If you have heart disease and are at high risk of cardiac arrhythmias—irregular heartbeats—that can trigger sudden death, you should be sure to get sufficient fish oil. New research suggests that fish oil can help keep heart rhythms from going berserk.

About a quarter of a million Americans die suddenly each year when their hearts abruptly go into a fatal arrhythmia—or wildly irregular heartbeats. It happens because the electrical transmission of impulses that govern the rate or rhythm of the heartbeat goes haywire. Although it can strike anyone out of the blue, people who have had heart attacks are at especially high risk. Now, remarkable new research suggests that fish oil may be a marvelous medicine to help regulate heart rhythms, preventing fatal cardiac arrhythmias. Such a promising role for fish oil is entirely new. Although researchers have known for years that eating fatty fish helps prevent heart disease, and notably death from heart disease, it was thought that fish oil acted mostly by protecting the arteries against plaque buildup and by thinning the blood. Now researchers suspect that the most profound benefits from fish oil come from directly protecting the heart against electrical malfunction leading to sudden death.

Harvard emeritus professor of medicine Dr. Alexander Leaf explains that fish oil affects the electrical activity and "excitability" of heart cells, just as it does brain cells. In impressive studies, Dr. Leaf has shown that it is much more difficult to induce heart arrhythmias in dogs that are first given fish oil. Indeed, he consistently found it took a 50 percent stronger electrical stimulus to induce cardiac arrythmias in heart cells that contained high levels of omega-3 fatty acids. Dr. Leaf has new research under way to test the theory in humans. In his new study, patients with implanted defibrillators, who have already had heart attacks, will take either fish oil capsules or a placebo dummy pill for a year. The study will reveal whether fish oil reduces the number of times the defibrillator must discharge to correct a heart arrhythmia.

At least two major studies, in England and France, tend to indirectly confirm the therapeutic ability of omega-3 fat to suppress fatal arrhythmias after a heart attack. In studies of about 1,600 patients, those who ate omega-3 as fatty fish, fish oil capsules, or canola oil were much less apt to suffer subsequent fatal heart attacks (not necessarily nonfatal heart attacks) than those not taking in high omega-3. In fact, in one study not a single patient on high omega-3s died of cardiac arrest. Also, direct support for the idea comes from a new study in Denmark of fifty-five heart attack patients. Half took fish oil capsules (5 grams or about 15 capsules a day) for three months. The fish oil affected their hearts in ways that inhibited deadly cardiac arrhythmias.

What's most remarkable, says Dr. Leaf, is that omega-3 "medication" appears to give rapid protection against cardiac sudden death. Researchers have noticed a reduction in cardiac deaths within a month of increased intakes of omega-3 fatty acids. Compare that with the two or three years needed to reap the heart attack protection of lowering your blood cholesterol. This newly discovered direct effect of omega-3s on heart function also helps explain why fish eaters have fewer heart attacks and are less apt to die from them.

Further, new evidence reveals that fish oil, like vitamin C, influences all-important "vascular function," keeping arteries more relaxed and open so blood can flow through. The omega-3s, like the vitamin, somehow trigger release of nitric oxide, the chemical that tells artery walls to relax.

Certainly anyone who has ever had a heart attack—or who has signs of heart disease—should seriously consider fish oil an essential medication that could be lifesaving, particularly by suppressing deadly fibrillation, if a heart attack occurs.

IT SMASHES TRIGLYCERIDES

Fish oil can curb heart disease in other ways. In fact, it is almost a sure cure—*better than any known drug*—for high tryglycerides, a type of blood fat that can be dangerous to arteries, especially when coupled with low good-type HDL cholesterol. In fact, fish oil is probably the safest and best "drug" around for reducing triglycerides, according to a new analysis of the data by William Harris, Ph.D., director of the Lipoprotein Research Laboratory, Mid America Heart Institute of St. Luke's Hospital, in Kansas City. Dr. Harris reviewed seventy-two well-controlled human studies and found that fish oil supplements reduced abnormally high triglycerides an average of 28 percent in patients. The effective fish oil dose was 3,000 to 4,000 milligrams daily, which is ten to thirteen capsules of the 300-milligram capsules commonly available in health food stores. New high-potency fish oil capsules are in the works, which would cut the number down to three or four capsules and would be sold through pharmacies. You can count on fish oil to work quickly; triglycerides start to sink in a few days and hit normal within a couple of weeks.

A possible drawback: Fish oil typically raises bad LDL cholesterol slightly, discouraging some doctors from recommending the oil to reduce triglycerides. Dr. Harris does not find this worrisome, but Canadian researchers have come up with a solution: Also take garlic. In a recent study, when men took 900 milligrams of garlic powder daily along with fish oil capsules, triglycerides fell 34 percent and LDL cholesterol dropped 9.5 percent. The senior author, Bruce J. Holub of the University of Guelph in Ontario, urges trying "effective and safe" combination before resorting to expensive prescription drugs to lower triglycerides and cholesterol.

The triglyceride-lowering alternative: very high doses of niacin or prescription drugs, all with potentially hazardous side effects.

It Relieves Arthritis Pain

The number one, best-tested natural "remedy of choice" to relieve the symptoms of rheumatoid arthritis is omega-3 fish oil. More than a dozen well-conducted studies over the last ten years show that consuming fish oil helps relieve the pain, swelling, and stiffness of rheumatoid arthritis, according to leading authority Dr. Joel Kremer, head of rheumatology at the Albany Medical College in New York. In one Belgian study, taking 2.6 grams of omega-3s fish oil daily not only reduced pain and strengthened hand grip but enabled almost half the subjects to decrease their doses of NSAID painkillers.

The doses needed to attain relief are fairly high—from 3,000 to 5,000 milligrams of omega-3s a day, says Dr. Kremer. Fish oil capsules in pharmacies and health food stores generally contain 300 milligrams. It's easy to figure: That means ten to seventeen capsules a day. Dr. Kremer says you generally should take the fish oil continuously for at least twelve weeks before expecting improvement. The improvement is greater for most people after eighteen to twenty-four weeks.

The oils work by manipulating the inflammatory process within cells. For example, tests show that fish oil suppresses the production of specific leukotrienes, agents that fire up inflammation.

GREAT MEDICINE FOR COLITIS

Especially exciting is new research on the use of fish oil to treat inflammatory bowel diseases, including Crohn's disease and ulcerative colitis. One of the pioneers in this treatment is William Stenson, M.D., at Washington University Medical Center in St. Louis. In one controlled study of eighteen patients, Dr. Stenson found that fish oil supplements slashed inflammatory agents called leukotriene B4, present in the colon, by an astonishing 60 percent. Typically, the more of these inflammatory agents, the more severe the disease. As expected, patients felt much better and gained weight, and examinations by sigmoidoscopy revealed less inflammation and damage. Further, the dosage of prednisone, a steroid drug, needed to keep the disease under control in seven patients dropped by more than half.

In other research Italian investigators have saved Crohn's patients from relapse by giving them fish oil. In a study of seventy-eight Crohn's patients at high risk of relapse, half were given nine specially coated fish oil capsules daily, the others dummy pills. After a year 59 percent on the fish oil were in remission compared with 26 percent on placebo. The study, as reported in the *New England Journal of Medicine* in 1996, used special "enteric-coated" fish capsules that were preferable because they disintegrated in the colon in an hour and did not taste fishy. Fish oil "seems to be one of the truly nontoxic medications to give to patients [in remission] on a long-term basis to prevent relapse," said Albert B. Knapp, assistant professor of medicine at New York University's School of Medicine.

The Safety Factor

If you want to try large doses of fish oil capsules therapeutically, be sure to check with your doctor first if you are also on other medications, especially anticoagulants, or have any serious disease or disorder. Fish oil does prolong bleeding time, although Harvard's Dr. Leaf says it is not as profound as generally thought. He points out that studies using ten grams of fish oil given with aspirin did not have a significant pro-bleeding effect. However, it is best to consult your doctor about any possible medication interactions with fish oil.

Further, high doses of fish oil can damage immune functioning unless you counteract the risk by taking 400 IU to 800 IU of vitamin E a day, according to Tufts University researchers.

How Much Do You Need?

The precise dose of omega–3s needed to ward off heart attacks is not known, although much research indicates that most healthy people can probably can get enough omega–3 to their hearts and arteries by eating oily fish, such as salmon, mackerel, sardines, herring, and anchovies two or three times a week. However, if you don't like fish, can't eat that much, have had a heart attack, or are at high risk of heart disease, or need therapeutic doses, fish oil capsules are the answer. Indeed, some researchers think most Americans could benefit from taking one or two standard fish oil capsules a day—a dose of 300 to 600 milligrams of omega–3 fatty acids, to fight artery-clogging and possibly prevent heart stoppage. Some capsules now have a higher content of omega–3s (EPA and DHA), so check the label.

Consumer Concerns
Some fears have been expressed over the possibility of excessive oxidation (cell-destroying free radicals) and environmental contaminants, such as pesticides and mercury, in fish oil capsules. However, Harvard's Dr. Leaf, who takes fish oil capsules himself, says he considers the capsules safe, in fact, safer than eating certain fish, for example, those from contaminated waters. He says responsible processors do meticulously "cleanse" the fish oils to be put in capsules of hazardous agents and add vitamin E to inhibit oxidation. (Be sure the capsule contains vitamin E, which will be noted on the label.) One way to determine a good quality pure fish oil capsule, says one industry expert, is by the light color of the oil. He suggests laying different brands of fish oil capsules on a white piece of paper and choosing the capsule that appears lightest.

One brand of fish oil capsule that has been widely used in research is MaxEpa. Another company that has a particularly good reputation within the industry for producing high-quality, pure fish oil capsules is General Nutrition Corporation.

Caution: Always store fish oil capsules, or any capsules of vegetable oils, in the refrigerator. Lower temperatures can slow down the rate at which they turn rancid; rancidity is the same as oxidation, or the generation of dangerous free radical chemicals that promote all types of chronic diseases.

Important: Too much of a type of fat called omega–6 can sabotage the benefits of fish oil. This omega–6 fat is found in vegetable oils, primarily corn oil, regular safflower and sunflower seed oil, and products made with them, such as mayonnaise, shortenings, and salad oils. Animal fat in meat and dairy foods can also overwhelm the omega-3 fat in cells, throwing things out of whack. To get the full benefit of fish oil, in food or capsules, you must also cut down on animal fats and omega–6 fats.

WHY NOT COD LIVER OIL?

Although some people report that their rheumatism is relieved by cod liver oil, such oil is not a substitute for omega-3 fish oil in treating disease. As the name implies, cod liver oil comes from the liver of the fish, and it does not actually contain high levels of beneficial omega-3s. The high omega-3 oil put in capsules comes from the whole body of the fish, such as mackerel, menhaden, and halibut, and is processed to have specific amounts of EPA and DHA fatty acids. Also, too much cod liver oil can be dangerous. Cod liver oil, unless it has been stripped of vitamin A and D, is very high in these fat-soluble vitamins, which can build up in the body and become toxic.

Prostate "Remedy of Choice"

(SAW PALMETTO)

It's at least as good as common prescription drugs and will probably leave you a whole lot happier.

If you're a man over age fifty, the chances are fifty-fifty that you have an enlarged prostate, medically known as benign prostatic hyperplasia (BPH), and the odds escalate as you grow older. It's no picnic. A swollen prostate gland, typically two to three times normal size, can squeeze your urethra, interfering with normal urination. Symptoms range from annoying—getting up frequently at night to urinate—to serious: pain from obstruction of urinary flow and trouble with erections. It is a nonmalignant condition.

You can cure it several ways. You can have surgery, which is very effective but carries the risk of incontinence or impotence. You can take prescription drugs that may or may not work but can also depress your libido and make you impotent. You can try various therapies, such as laser or microwave, to zap or vaporize unwanted prostate tissue. You can just "watch and wait," as some physicians advise, to avoid drugs and surgery as long as possible. You may also get rid of the symptoms by taking a berry extract, a successful treatment widely used in Europe, that costs about one-third as much as conventional drugs and has virtually no risk of side effects. It has worked for millions of men.

JON'S MIRACLE
The Pain Is Gone, the Sex Is Back

Jonathan Weil* had it all—good fortune and good health. At age fifty-eight he was a successful Chicago attorney and businessman with a new second wife and blood pressure most younger men would envy; he was so trim he weighed the same as he had in college—and he never took pills, including aspirin, because he was never sick, not even with an occasional headache.

But then this nagging problem began to intrude on his peace of mind. He first noticed it in the men's john. "You go to a washroom and the younger guys have a strong stream," he says "and yours is sort of, well, not trickling, but it's not what it used to be. Even my nine-year-old grandson had a stream that sounded like Niagara Falls next to me." More disturbing, his manhood was fading away; his erections were much weaker, and he worried about sexual failure with his new wife.

Since his two brothers, one a physician, had complained of enlarged prostate, he was aware of the problem, so he consulted a urologist, then another and another, who all agreed: "That's what comes with age." Now for the hard part. He considered joining a double-blind study of the drug

Proscar, but backed out when he learned of one side effect—"It lessens your erection."

Then he heard about Dr. Glenn Gerber, a urologist at Chicago Medical Center, who was testing saw palmetto for enlarged prostate. Dr. Gerber became interested because so many of his patients were enthusiastically using the botanical medicine on their own, having read about it in health magazines. Dr. Gerber's study is exceptional in that he uses sophisticated techniques to measure benefit, such as pressure within the bladder. Reduced size of the prostate, he says, does not always mean improvement in symptoms.

Jon Weil began taking two capsules of saw palmetto daily, the same stuff you get in any health food store. He hoped to see improvement in a month, but it was more like three months. "Then all of a sudden, my God, what an improvement in the stream!" It wasn't 100 percent strong all the time, but enough to make him happy. Most of all, he was ecstatic about the return of his strong erections. "Sex is renewed all of a sudden," he says. Side effects? None at all.

Dr. Gerber's six-month study is not over, but he says many men, like Weil, "have had marked improvement in their symptoms. Others feel the stuff did little or nothing, which is true of any therapy." And a statistical analysis of the results, including the bladder-pressure tests, will not be done until the study is complete. Still, Dr. Gerber says, many of the patients, including Weil, plan to continue on saw palmetto because they're sure it helped. The key question: Would the expert physician Dr. Gerber take saw palmetto if he had BPH?

Yes, he says. "There's very little downside to it, so I don't think people have a lot to lose by trying it. It may do a lot of good, and in the worst case scenario, it does no harm."

*A pseudonym has been used to protect privacy, but the medical details are accurate.

What Is It?

The herbal extract is processed from the brownish-black berries of the saw palmetto plant, a smallish member of the fan palm family that grows mainly in the southeastern United States. The plant has long been used to treat prostate troubles. Until the mid-twentieth century, saw palmetto was listed in the National Formulary of the United States as a treatment for enlarged prostate. Now the berries are shipped to Europe, where they are processed by pharmaceutical companies into pills and extracts. Then they are sent back to the United States and sold as a "dietary supplement" because the FDA forbids calling them a medication.

What's the Evidence?

The evidence for saw palmetto is impressive, despite a confounding factor in research that finds any BPH treatment has a strong "placebo effect" of as much as 30 to 40 percent, some contend. That means much of the perceived benefit of a test drug is "all in the mind"; an inactive pill, called a placebo, might do as well. However, from a sufferer's point of view, if saw palmetto does work partly in the psyche, it is a much cheaper, safer "sugar pill" than pharmaceuticals (such as Proscar), which also have the same strong placebo effect but can have side effects that can do more harm than the drug does good.

Research on saw palmetto has been sufficient to merit the scientific approval and status among physicians that make it a best-seller in Europe. Around twenty human studies credit the herbal medicine with as much as a 90 percent success rate in treating enlarged prostate. That's more cure power than pharmaceutical drugs and surgery can boast. Some studies were short-term and did not account for a placebo effect. But of seven well-conducted (double-blind placebo) studies on saw palmetto extract, six deemed the plant superior to a dummy pill after one to three months of use.

For example, saw palmetto had a super effect in a study of 110 men with enlarged prostate who were given either the herbal medicine or a dummy pill, as reported in the *British Journal of Clinical Pharmacology* in 1984. Saw palmetto extract in a dose of 320 milligrams a day worked ten times better than the placebo at improving urine flow rates. It was about five times more effective than the dummy pill in promoting emptying of the bladder. The saw palmetto takers also did not have to get up at night to urinate as often; nor did they experience as much pain, discomfort, or difficulty in urinating as they had before taking the plant extract. Further, all these benefits happened within thirty days!

A typical and convincing study of thirty men by Italian investigators in 1983 found similar improvements from saw palmetto. After one month on the plant extract, men's urine flow rates increased dramatically, exceeding any benefits from placebo by seventeenfold.

In large "open" tests without placebo, saw palmetto is also heralded by its users. In 1993 German investigators gave saw palmetto extract to 1,334 patients for six months. Eighty percent rated the treatment "good to excellent." Frequency of urination decreased 37 percent, nighttime urination sank 54 percent, and ability to empty the bladder increased 50 percent.

In a more recent "open" study at several medical centers in Belgium involving 305 patients, saw palmetto produced even more remarkable success, as judged by physicians, patients, and objective measurements. After three months 88 percent of the patients said their symptoms were reduced and they felt their quality of life was better; notably, their sleep was not disturbed as frequently by urges to get up and urinate. The physicians agreed with the overall 88 percent effectiveness of the remedy. Rigorous measurements by standard tests also verified the therapy. For example, urine flow rates increased 25 percent; prostate size decreased 10 percent. And most important, scores on a well-respected international prostate symptom test dropped 35 percent.

How Does It Work?

It's not clear exactly how saw palmetto works. The most common theory is that saw palmetto reduces levels of a very active form of the male hormone testosterone known as dihydrotestosterone or DHT, thought to be the primary spur to enlargement of the prostate. It's a weird situation. An enzyme switches on the DHT, fooling the cells into thinking they are in puberty again and need to get going. So the DHT causes an overproduction of prostate cells, causing the gland to grow bigger. Men with enlarged prostate have exceptionally high levels of DHT; so do men with prostate cancer. Specifically, studies show that saw palmetto extract blocks the action of the enzyme that instigates production of DHT. In other words, it is a hormone suppressor.

What are the active agents in saw palmetto? Many experts credit plant sterols, mainly sitosterol. It has hormonal effects as well as antiinflammatory activity and may directly inhibit growth of prostate cells. Many believe a combination of compounds working together account for saw palmetto's therapeutic action.

How Much Do You Need?
The recommended dose, found effective in studies, is 320 milligrams of standardized extract a day, taken all at once or in two doses.

How Quickly Does It Work?
Surprisingly, studies find that saw palmetto can bring rapid relief—within twenty-eight days, according to one study that used 320 milligrams daily. Compare that with the drug Proscar, which usually does not produce noticeable benefits until taken for six months to a year. However, the benefits of saw palmetto usually accumulate, so using it longer predicts greater improvement. Nationally recognized naturopathic doctor Donald Brown of Seattle advises his patients to take 320 milligrams of saw palmetto daily for at least four to six weeks to see if it's working. If so, count on its being a part of your life from then on, he says.

The Safety Factor
What makes saw palmetto popular with doctors and other health practitioners is the virtual lack of side effects and toxicity. A few cases of stomach upset and intestinal bloating have been reported. As far as anyone knows, no acute or long-term toxicity exists. Nor is there evidence of interactions with prescription drugs.

Should You Try It?
If you lived in Germany, it's almost sure your doctor would prescribe saw palmetto, perhaps along with other

plant remedies. Saw palmetto is approved for benign prostatic hyperplasia (BPH) in Germany. Indeed, according to
a 1993 report, a whopping 90 percent of patients with
BPH in Germany are given plant medicinals, and 50 percent of German urologists prefer the plant extracts to
chemically derived pharmaceuticals. Of all plants, saw
palmetto is most widely used, sometimes as a main ingredient combined with other plant extracts.

Caution: It's not wise to self-diagnose BPH. If you have
prostate symptoms, see a doctor, because the symptoms
might indicate other problems, including a treatable cancer. Before trying saw palmetto or other herbal treatment,
you must have a medical diagnosis of BPH. Even then it is
advisable to use the herb under the supervision of a health
professional.

SAW PALMETTO OR PROSCAR?

If you are offered the prescription drug finasteride, better
known as Proscar, very popular for treating BPH, here are
some facts you should know. Proscar has significant side
effects, especially on male sexual function, says Ralph
Nader's Health Research Group. One of twenty men who
take it experiences impotence and one out of sixteen has
decreased libido, the group says, concluding that taking
Proscar, unless you really have to, is a bad idea. Further,
the drug may not work any better than a dummy pill,
according to a 1996 study of 1,229 men that compared
Proscar with both a placebo and another newly approved
drug for BPH, Abbott's Hytrin. After one year Proscar was
judged ineffective, no better than a placebo in treating
BPH, according to Herbert Lepor, chief of urology at New
York University Medical Center, who headed the study.
(Hytrin was better than either Proscar or placebo.) Merck,
the maker of Proscar, called the study flawed.

Commenting on the study, Dr. H. Logan Holtgrewe, a past president of the American Urological Association, lamented the high treatment failure for BPH that sends frustrated men from one ineffective treatment to another, driving up the health care costs. "The cascading effect leads to much greater costs than if you had gone to [the best] treatment to begin with."

Actually, saw palmetto should be a man's first choice, says Dr. Michael Murray of Seattle, a nationally recognized naturopathic doctor and author of many books, including *Natural Alternatives to Over-the-Counter and Prescription Drugs*. His reasons: Proscar is effective in less than 37 percent of patients; it takes six months to a year to produce significant improvement; and it has serious sexually related side effects. In contrast, saw palmetto is effective in almost 90 percent of men; it works much more quickly, within four to six weeks, and it has no side effects or toxicity. Proscar costs about three times as much—$75 compared with saw palmetto's $24 a month.

SAW PALMETTO PLUS
Saw palmetto may work even better when mixed with other herbs. Some researchers in Europe and the United States are now testing a combination of saw palmetto with other herbs—pygeum, pumpkin seed, and stinging nettle root extract. One product called Prostagutt Forte™, combining saw palmetto and stinging nettle root, in Germany has been highly effective, in many cases better than saw palmetto alone. A U.S. product called Pros-Forte (Vitaline Corporation), which is a mixture of 160 milligrams of saw palmetto, 50 milligrams of pygeum, and 100 milligrams of pumpkin seed, also tested well recently.

In the study Dr. Stuart I. Erner, board-certified internist at Albany Memorial Hospital in New York, gave two tablets of Pros-Forte daily to twenty men with documented prostate disorders—either BPH or chronic intermittent prostatitis. Fully 90 percent had improvement of symptoms, ranging in a reduction of symptoms from 12 percent to 79 percent, as judged by standard test measures. Nearly all reported improvement after four weeks of treatment. Dr. Erner notes that those with the most severe symptoms improved the most. None experienced serious side effects, he says.

Surprising Gout Medicines

(CELERY AND CHERRY EXTRACTS)

If you have gout, check out these two folk remedies. There's no firm scientific evidence that they
work, but there are a lot of people who say they
do. And some scientists are taking a new look at
them.

If you have gout, you know what it is and how painful it
can be. For those who do not suffer its torment, gout is a
form of arthritis involving sudden attacks in joints that
can cause intense pain, swelling, and redness, lasting perhaps a few hours but usually a few days. Sometimes the
pain is nearly constant because of chronic inflammation.
Most often stricken is the big toe, but the knees, ankle,
wrist, foot, and small joints of the hand are also affected. If
uncontrolled, gout can lead to serious kidney disease. It is
characterized by high blood levels of uric acid that crystal-
lize in the joints, causing extreme pain and inflammation.
Usual treatment is high doses of NSAIDS (painkillers) and
drugs, such as allopurinol, that inhibit formation of uric
acid. Gout is sometimes jokingly called the "arthritis of
geniuses and kings" because it afflicted people such as Ben
Franklin and King Henry VIII.

THE DOCTOR'S DILEMMA

Before your doctor will tell you to take cherry juice or celery seed for your gout, he or she will probably want some scientific evidence on them. Frankly, there just aren't any real, hard, modern-type data that these plant medicines work, or how they work, or how often they work. But that does not bother some believers in tradition who think that just the fact that they have been used for years as folk remedies constitutes persuasive evidence in itself.

As much as we desire pharmacological explanations to persuade us that a particular substance is valid, sometimes the only thing that makes it valid is human experience. In medical lingo, that is called "anecdotal," and cuts little ice with medical purists who want hard proof that it works not just for a few individuals, but for the general population as determined by tests in people chosen at random—and, further, that it works better statistically than a so-called placebo or sugar pill in subjects who don't know which they are taking. But when you are the person for whom the cure works, it works 100 percent, and you may not care whether the relief comes from a placebo effect or whether the remedy also works in a certain percentage of other people—whether hundreds of others have had the same relief.

In that spirit of nearly pure "anecdote," with little or no understanding at present of why they might work, here are a couple of botanical remedies that many people have tried and raved about as "miracle" cures for gout. Indeed, a new folklore is emerging over such remedies, along with a new scientific interest. Whether research will validate and explain these popular remedies is unknown.

THE CHERRY JUICE CURE

It's uncertain exactly how the whole thing got started, but the cherry juice cure may have originated in modern times with a fellow named Ludwig Blau, Ph.D., who in 1950 wrote an article entitled "Cherry Diet Control for Gout and Arthritis" in the *Texas Reports on Biology and Medicine*. He described how he had cured his crippling gout, which had confined him to a wheelchair, by eating six to eight cherries every day. Continuing to eat cherries, he claimed, kept painful gout away. He also cited twelve others who had cured their gout by eating cherries or drinking cherry juice. Soon afterward *Prevention* magazine added to the mystery and mystique by publishing Dr. Blau's advice to use cherries as gout medicine. Dozens of gout victims wrote in to testify that eating cherries—fifteen to twenty-five a day initially and ten a day afterward as a maintenance dose—had relieved their suffering and pain.

Dr. Blau admitted he had no scientific reason to explain why cherries worked. Neither does anyone else, apparently. Searches of the medical literature found no studies confirming it and no medically plausible theories to explain why it should work. Nor are there clues as to which constituents of the cherry juice might have pharmacological activity. Nevertheless, the practice has persisted, and many people still swear it does work, claiming as much relief from cherry juice as from commonly prescribed antigout drugs that can have troubling side effects. But now you don't have to depend on plain old cherry juice in the grocery store; you can buy concentrated cherry juice in liquid or capsule form at health food stores. Popular thought holds that black cherries, especially in the form of black cherry juice concentrate, are far better than red cherries. But all of this is modern folk medicine in the making.

BRAD'S MIRACLE
No More Pain, No More Drugs

Gout was ruining his life, and Brad McAdams, a forty-four-year-old draftsman in an oil refinery in Corpus Christi, Texas, was worried. Diagnosed about seven years earlier, the gout had become so painful—primarily in his knees, but also in his ankles—that he could barely walk. "It really hurt to move. There would be times when I just couldn't get out of bed." Nor did he sleep well, because of the intense pain. Sometimes he limped badly and could no longer walk through the plant on his job. When the barometric pressure fell in wintertime, triggering flare-ups of gout, he became virtually confined to his office chair. It was also difficult for him to share his love of archery with his two young daughters. After standing in place shooting at a target, he could barely walk to retrieve the arrows because "my leg was so stiff."

It was a classic case of gout, confirmed by high uric acid levels in Brad's blood. Naturally his doctor had prescribed the appropriate drugs: allopurinol to relieve the recurrent attacks by blocking formation of uric acid, and indomethacin for pain. When the pain and swelling were unbearable, his doctor injected painkilling cortisone into the joints.

The drugs helped, especially the cortisone, which usually stopped the pain instantly; but still the gout attacks came back. And McAdams hated the side effects. "The pain medication the doctor gave me was so strong it made me go to sleep." He also became alarmed when his eyesight worsened, and his doctor found "strange" blood changes, suggesting leukemia. Brad even had a bone marrow test in search of a cause. He feared it was all a side effect of the allopurinol.

So when his mother-in-law called from Alabama to say she had seen a television show about a natural remedy for gout—black cherry juice concentrate—he was definitely up for trying it. He started taking two tablespoons of the concentrate at night. It tasted terrible, he says, but he kept it up, and after a couple of weeks his attacks of gout stopped. By the end of the month, in December 1994, he stopped taking his prescription medicines, and has not taken them since. "He's back to normal," says his wife. "He hasn't had a flare-up of gout for two years." He still takes the black cherry concentrate liquid—not the newer pills that are available—occasionally, mostly in winter when he fears attacks of gout. "It works; it really does," he says. His present doctor confirms that he no longer prescribes antigout drugs for Brad, and as far as he knows, his patient no longer has acute attacks of gout. Was it the black cherry juice extract? "It's possible," his doctor grants.

DR. DUKE'S MIRACLE
"I Didn't Believe It at First"

Probably nobody on the face of the earth knows more about medicinal plants than James Duke,

Ph.D., a medical botanist formerly with the U.S. Department of Agriculture. He has designed databases of the pharmacological activity of plants and plant chemicals. He has written learned, scholarly books on the subject that are studied by other experts, as well as popular articles and books. One other thing: Jim suffers from gout. "I had my first attack of gout when I was forty-seven," he says, "I'm now sixty-seven, so it's twenty years ago." Typically the first "crisis," as it's called, was in his big toe. He had many more extremely painful attacks. Reluctantly, ten years ago, he started taking allopurinol to reduce high blood levels of uric acid. Through the years he has tried various herbal remedies, including cherry juice, but they didn't really work for him, so he stayed on the prescription drug.

Then in July 1996 he saw an ad in a new magazine *Herbs for Health*, for a gout remedy he had never heard of—celery seed extract. "Now I've heard a lot about celery, but I've never heard that it's hypouremic—lowers uric acid. That was the pitch in the ad," says Duke. "So I wrote and said I don't believe it, but I'm willing to give it the college try and there's nobody better to experiment on than me." That's because Jim knows that if he does certain things, like drink "a six-pack of cheap beer when I'm on one of my Amazon jungle trips," he is sure to pay dearly with a gout attack if he's not on allopurinol.

So he stopped taking the drug cold turkey in July and started taking celery seed tablets, at first four a day. "I figured I would surely have an attack, but it never happened. It was a week, two weeks, three weeks. I said, Hey, maybe there's something to this." Since then he has gone on several field trips to the Amazon to study wild plants, where one time he did down "a six-pack of cheap beer." Another time he even seriously threw his hip out of joint while "dancing vigorously on the banks of the Amazon. That surely would have triggered an attack of gout without allopurinol, but I was on the celery seed then. I'm delighted to say I've been off allopurinol for seven months and taking celery seed extract and it's working." He has not had a single attack of gout since he started the celery seed extract. He now takes two tablets daily.

What might account for celery seed's powers? "Well, there's some weak evidence in the medical literature from Australia and South Africa," he says. But what surprised him most was what he found on celery seed in his own extensive database, now administered by the Department of Agriculture. "I went to the database and saw something new, that celery seed contains about twenty different antiinflammatory agents. Maybe that helps explain it."

Dr. Duke doesn't know whether celery seed lowers his uric acid, as the ad claims, because he hasn't yet had it measured. However, to make his experience more than "anecdotal," he favors clinical testing to find out what is happening and how well celery seed extract may work on others with gout.

As far as anyone knows, the only medical test of celery seed was a small study of eight arthritis sufferers by Brian Daunter, Ph.D., at the University of Queensland in Australia. The volunteers took celery seed extract for six weeks, and about half reported less pain as rated by a special questionnaire. When they stopped taking the celery seed, they said the pain returned. The most pain relief occurred after twelve weeks, the researcher noted.

THE AUSTRALIAN CELERY CRAZE

Actually, celery seed has long been used as a traditional folk medicine in England and Australia to treat arthritis of various types, says Kerry Bone, leading expert on herbal remedies and technical director of MediHerb, Australia's largest pharmaceutical maker of herbal medicines. Bone says a craze for celery seed to treat arthritis a few years ago in Australia depleted the commercial supply of the herb. Although scientific evidence is lacking, he suspects celery seed works because of its anti-inflammatory activity, and possibly because it helps remove uric acid from the body, which is a rationale given by traditional herbal practitioners. Celery seed, he says, is an excellent example of an herb that "has no modern scientific data but works brilliantly in patients." So promising is celery seed that a new research institute affiliated with Australia's University of Queensland is establishing a center to do extensive research on the antiarthritic activity of celery seed.

The Safety Factor
No side effects have been reported for either concentrated cherry juice or celery seed extracts, although allergic reactions are always possible. Long-term toxicity is not much of a concern, because these substances have been used as food for centuries.

Who Should Not Take It?
Women who are pregnant or people with kidney disease should avoid celery seed because of its potential diuretic effect.

Consumer Concerns

The celery seed product used by Dr. Duke is CelereX, developed in Australia. It costs about $10 for sixty tablets and is available in some retail stores and by mail order at 800–792–2830. Cherry juice extract is widely available in health food stores.

Should You Try It?

If for some reason your current gout treatment is not effective or you want to get off certain painkillers or antigout drugs, these two gout folk remedies may be worth a try. However, Dr. Duke admits he disobeyed doctor's orders by stopping allopurinol abruptly, but says that he was willing to bet on celery seed extract and suffer the consequences if it didn't work. It's highly doubtful that cherry juice or celery seed extracts will work for everyone. (Neither do pharmaceutical drugs.) It's always best to consult your doctor or another health professional before dropping prescription medications or lowering doses.

New Answer to Chronic Fatigue Puzzle

(LICORICE)

The root can hurt most of us, but that's exactly why it might help cure baffling "incurable" chronic fatigue syndrome.

If someone could find a cure or partial cure for a perplexing, virtually untreatable disorder known as chronic fatigue syndrome, it would end much misery for many throughout the world. Chronic fatigue syndrome, also known as CFS, may not be what you think. It's not a normal state of tiredness. Sure, you may get tired, exhausted at times, but that's not CFS. CFS is characterized by a cluster of symptoms that often defies diagnosis and treatment. Suddenly a healthy, vital person is struck by a prolonged flulike illness, accompanied by headaches, joint and muscle pain, depression, and, most of all, unrelenting intense fatigue that may keep a person away from work and in bed all day—all from no apparent cause. When doctors can put no other name to it, they label it chronic fatigue syndrome. But nobody really knows how to treat it (common therapy: painkillers and antidepressants) or what causes it; recovery is rare and frustration is high.

As *Consumer Reports* magazine recently observed: "Probably hundreds of thousands of people in the U.S. have chronic fatigue syndrome. . . . Theories about the cause cover just about everything, including hormonal, immunological, and neurological abnormalities. The ailment is every bit as baffling as it is devastating."

Now comes the intriguing possibility that this most perplexing and debilitating malady might be relieved by one of nature's oldest medicines—licorice root. As new research emerges defining some of the poorly understood mechanisms behind chronic fatigue syndrome, some experts and patients find the pharmacological activity of licorice perfectly suited to the treatment of the disorder. However, licorice is not appropriate for everyone with chronic fatigue, and in some cases could actually make you worse. It's important to use it with caution, preferably with the advice and supervision of a health professional. But when chronic fatigue is due to specific biochemical deficiencies—mainly a type of low blood pressure—licorice, a uniquely effective and relatively benign drug, compared with conventional pharmaceutical interventions, could help pull off a "miracle" cure, as it has done for others.

DAVE'S MIRACLE
"I Felt Fantastic for the First Time in Twenty Years"

For David Williams, also known as Captain Dave, now age fifty-five and a longtime captain of fishing and charter boats in southern Florida, it began in 1977 as it does typically, with an overwhelming fatigue, following a severe chest cold. "I was so absolutely tired and exhausted, you know, bone-tired and unable to think because of brain fog." He recalls being unable to make it from the garage to the house without sitting down. "I just felt, What the hell is wrong with me?"

Also typically, his condition was not readily diagnosed. His life became a nightmare during the next years; he lost several businesses, jobs, and his wife. "The mental fog, the fatigue, everything just sort of crashed in on me." He saw "doctor after doctor after doctor," including several counselors and psychiatrists. "One tried me on all kinds of different psychiatric drugs, but nothing worked." He was in despair. "I just knew I wasn't going to get better." On the verge of total breakdown, he went to a local VA hospital (he is a veteran). "I just threw myself on their mercy. I said, God, you've got to help me. You've got to find out what's wrong with me. Why am I so bloody fatigued all the time?" They referred him to immunologists at the University of Miami; there in 1992 he was given the diagnosis of chronic fatigue syndrome. But it didn't help much, nor did the typical trial-and-error treatment. He did not feel a great deal better.

Then in late 1995—breakthrough. For the first time doctors at Johns Hopkins found that some chronic fatigue is caused by a type of low blood pressure abnormality. Williams was referred to Dr. Marilyn Cox, then at the University of Miami, for a "tilt table test" that definitively identifies the low blood pressure disorder. If you pass out rather quickly after being suspended upright on the tilt table, you have it. He did. Bingo. The next obvious step: Boost blood pressure. His doctors prescribed the drug fludrocortisone (Florinef), which causes salt and fluid retention and raises blood pressure and blood volume. By raising blood pressure, the theory goes, the drug could also indirectly erase symptoms of chronic fatigue syndrome by increasing the circulation of blood and oxygen to the brain. But Williams had a bad reaction to it and similar drugs.

Still on a quest, Williams started his own research at his local library. By plugging into the National Library of Medicine's Medline, he discovered two letters to the editor of the *New Zealand Medical Journal* from an Italian physician, Dr. Riccardo Baschetti, reporting how he had cured his own chronic fatigue by taking licorice. The reason: In some people licorice raises blood pressure. At first Williams scoffed. "I laughed. It was so utterly ridiculous to me." Nevertheless he contacted Dr. Baschetti, got his advice, and started taking licorice—about 4 grams daily. Williams was ecstatic: "I really felt fantastic. I mean, I just felt cured. Totally. One hundred percent. Brand new. I was so excited, I was amazed. I had been running around looking for this for twenty years, and blink, I get it."

As proof that licorice cured the abnormally low blood pressure, in turn alleviating the chronic fatigue symptoms, Williams retook the critical tilt table test in August 1996. If he survived without getting dizzy or fainting, it would mean his blood pressure abnormality was under control. "I passed with flying colors," he says. That's true, says Dr. Cox, a cardiologist now at Tallahassee Memorial

Regional Medical Center. She agrees that the licorice apparently normalized his blood pressure and in so doing, alleviated his chronic fatigue symptoms. "Scientifically it makes sense," she explains. "The main active ingredient in licorice, glycyrrhizinic acid, is a plant steroid that mimics the drug Florinef, prescribed to treat the low blood pressure abnormality." Dr. Cox, in fact, helped Williams experiment with different doses of licorice to find the exact one that normalized his blood pressure, enabling him to pass the tilt table test. She is writing up his case for a medical journal, and has heard of other chronic fatigue patients with low blood pressure taking licorice under the supervision of physicians.

What Is It?

Licorice, a member of the legume family, reportedly made its medical debut 5,000 years ago in China, being included in a compilation of herbal remedies called the Pen Tsao Ching.

Since then it has been used medicinally in ancient Egypt, in Greece, and in Europe in the Middle Ages and until the present day, mainly as a folk treatment for respiratory infections, colds, coughs, and more recently, ulcers. The part used is the root or rhizome. Today the roots are shredded, powdered, and made into black extracts, and licorice's principal active chemical, glycyrrhizic acid, has been isolated and is sometimes used separately.

What's the Evidence?

At first the idea that licorice could treat chronic fatigue may appear absurd to many people. But it takes on increasing credibility because of recent remarkable research presenting intriguing new explanations for the chronic fatigue puzzle and how it can be cleared up by drugs that work much the same way licorice does.

A landmark study at Johns Hopkins University that steered Dave Williams in the right direction was done by cardiologist Hugh Calkins and colleagues. They discovered that a startling 95 percent of twenty-three chronic fatigue sufferers—all but one—had a low blood pressure abnormality that can result in dilation of blood vessels and rapidly falling blood pressure, starving the brain of oxygen. Further, when Hopkins researchers gave the patients the drug fludrocortisone, which causes salt and fluid retention and raises blood pressure, the chronic fatigue symptoms disappeared completely or partially in nearly half of them.

Similarly, at the National Institutes of Health in 1991, Mark A. Demitrack and colleagues found that most chronic fatigue victims had a "mild adrenal insufficiency" that could help account for the hallmark symptoms of CFS, such as lethargy and fatigue, irregularities in immune response, and exaggerated allergic reactions. Amazingly, the governmental researchers concluded that the symptoms of chronic fatigue syndrome and this adrenal "insufficiency" were virtually identical! And how is this treated? With the drugs hydrocortisone and fludrocortisone, the same one that raised blood pressure and wiped out CFS symptoms in the Hopkins study.

In a nutshell: Many people with chronic fatigue syndrome may have a malfunctioning adrenal gland, resulting in so-called adrenal insufficiency—low levels of corticosteroids in the blood. This leads to abnormal excretion of minerals, particularly sodium, along with low blood pressure and low blood volume. Correcting the insufficiency with the proper steroids may relieve the symptoms of chronic fatigue.

And this is where licorice comes in. Licorice, in fact, is a natural steroid, with activity very similar to the powerful steroidal drug cortisone, says Italian physician Dr. Riccardo Baschetti, who uses licorice to treat his own chronic fatigue syndrome. Licorice, like steroidal drugs, can also raise blood pressure and cause fluid retention. Indeed, licorice eaters have long been warned to be aware of those specific harmful side effects. Ironically, the long-perceived negative pharmacological effect is what makes licorice a potential treatment for chronic fatigue.

Moreover, licorice was used medically in the 1950s to treat the classic "adrenal insufficiency" disorder known as Addison's disease. Dr. Baschetti believes that much chronic fatigue is in fact an atypical form of Addison's disease and should be treated as such. A new controlled study, sponsored by the National Institute of Allergy and Infectious Diseases, is under way to see if the drug fludro-cortisone (Florinef) does alleviate chronic fatigue syndrome by treating "adrenal insufficiency," for which it is commonly used. If so, it would also confirm the validity of licorice, which does much the same thing.

DR. BASCHETTI'S MIRACLE
"Licorice Revived My Stamina in a Few Days"

The Italian doctor's misery started abruptly on March 3, 1993, with "classic flulike symptoms." He worsened gradually, and "despite several pharmacological treatments, which all proved disappointingly ineffective, I was virtually bed-bound from

August to November 1993" with what was then diagnosed as chronic fatigue syndrome. Desperate, Dr. Riccardo Baschetti, a retired government health official, left his home in Padua and spent five weeks in Santo Domingo, hoping to recover in the tropical climate. He became even more ill. "The devastating effects of chronic fatigue syndrome have been generally underappreciated," he says. "It is indeed a serious illness."

Along with trying several drugs, Dr. Baschetti also tried changing his diet. To his utter surprise, he noted that eating salty foods made him feel better. Then it struck him that chronic fatigue syndrome might be an atypical form of adrenal insufficiency, similar to classic Addison's disease, in which there is a deficiency of aldosterone, the sodium-retaining hormone. He also remembered that licorice is "well-known primarily for its aldosteronelike effects and that until the 1950s, before cortisone became available, patients with Addison's disease were successfully treated with licorice."

Aha, he reasoned, if chronic fatigue is a hormonal insufficiency similar to Addison's disease, why wouldn't eating licorice help normalize the low hormone activity, thereby helping relieve his symptoms? He started eating licorice. For the first time in twenty months since his first attack of chronic fatigue, he noticed relief. "Licorice caused a revival of my physical and mental stamina within a few days!" Still he was not fully back to normal. He consumed more and more licorice, up to 30 grams, or about an ounce a day.

Then it dawned on him that dissolving the

licorice in sodium-rich milk might increase its potency. In October 1994 he dissolved 5 grams of solid extract of licorice in 1 liter of milk and drank it rapidly. "Shortly after, to my surprise, for about ten minutes I repeatedly breathed very deep sighs. Within two hours I felt virtually recovered." He now takes 4 grams of licorice a day dissolved in milk and very small amounts of a drug, hydrocortisone (2.5 milligrams daily), and continues to feel terrific. He attributes his complete recovery from chronic fatigue syndrome to licorice. Dr. Baschetti has spread the word of his experience and theories through reports and letters published in several prestigious medical journals. He says he relapsed only once when he stopped taking the licorice, as a test. "It's astonishingly effective," he says.

How Does It Work?

Licorice is one of nature's own corticosteroids, hormones produced by the adrenal glands, with pharmacological activity very similar to that of the powerful steroidal drug cortisone. Researchers have confirmed that the active agent in licorice that mimics cortisone is glycyrrhizinic acid. According to Dr. Baschetti, licorice's glycyrrhizinic acid works by blocking the activity of an enzyme (11 beta-hydroxysteroid dehydrogenase) that otherwise breaks down and destroys your own natural hormone, cortisol. Thus, by preserving more cortisol, licorice helps correct hormonal deficiencies common in both chronic fatigue and Addison's disease, he theorizes. Licorice, he says, imitates cortisone and other hormones that help regulate sodium retention and water balance.

Who Should Take It?

It's unclear how many people diagnosed with chronic fatigue have abnormally low blood pressure or adrenal insufficiency and thus might be helped by licorice. A clue comes from the Hopkins study: Researchers found that about half the subjects benefited from the drug, suggesting that the same percentage might be helped by licorice. On the other hand, the NIH study suggested that almost 70 percent of chronic fatigue sufferers may have "adrenal insufficiency" and might also benefit. Either figure is impressive, considering how few cures come with other treatments.

How Much Do You Need?

It depends on your body size. Since little has been published in mainstream medical journals on this matter, finding the right amount is often a matter of trial and error. That is why it is essential to be monitored by a doctor or another health professional if you try licorice to treat chronic fatigue syndrome or any other disorder. Some users have come up with their own doses. The dose that worked best for David Williams, after much trial and error, was 5 grams a day, containing 375 milligrams of glycyrrhizinic acid. This doesn't mean it's the right dose for everyone. (Williams is a big man, around 6-feet-2 and 240 pounds.) "Doses would probably need to be individualized and each patient carefully monitored by a doctor for results," says Dr. Cox.

Consumer Concerns

As a therapeutic agent, licorice must be the "real thing." Much of what Americans call licorice, used to flavor candies and sweets, is actually anise, not real licorice. Real licorice is available in health food stores as a powder and liquid extract. Some licorice has the glycyrrhizinic acid removed; since glycyrrhizinic acid is the agent that revs up cortisol output and retention of the critical natural steroid cortisol, licorice stripped of it would not work to relieve chronic fatigue syndrome. However, it is safer for normal people.

The Safety Factor

For normal people, eating licorice root in inappropriately high doses can have serious side effects, such as headache, lethargy, dangerously high blood pressure, and sodium and water retention (edema), possibly resulting in cardiac arrest and heart failure. Overdosing on licorice extract, or even candy, has caused hospitalizations. If you are using it for chronic fatigue syndrome, taking too much could also be a problem in upsetting potassium balance, which could precipitate heart failure. As for long-term toxicity, the Food and Drug Administration lists licorice root as generally regarded as safe (GRAS.)

Caution: Anyone taking licorice therapeutically, warns Dr. Cox, must be watched carefully for side effects, mainly depression of blood potassium to life-threatening low levels. Even though licorice is "natural," it is powerful and cannot be treated casually.

Who Should Not Take It?

People with high blood pressure, diabetes, glaucoma, heart disease, or a history of stroke and those on heart or blood pressure medications should not take licorice, nor should pregnant women. To be safe, always consult a doctor.

What Else Is It Good For?

Licorice is a longtime treatment for gastric ulcers. In Germany the government's authority on herbal medicines,

Commission E, approves the use of licorice to treat ulcers, recommending doses of 200 to 600 milligrams of glycyrrhizin daily (about 5 to 15 grams of root) for no longer than four to six weeks. Other research shows that licorice may also help fight viruses and boost immune functioning.

HOW TO USE LICORICE FOR CHRONIC FATIGUE
Advice and Cautions
from Dr. Riccardo Baschetti

Dr. Baschetti advises dissolving 2 grams of pure nondeglycyrrhinized licorice in about a pint of cold low-fat or skim milk. Use finely ground licorice and soak it for about twelve hours in a little water to make it dissolve more easily. Drink the beverage every morning. You should notice improvement in a few hours! If not, you can gradually and cautiously increase the dosage of licorice up to 5 grams in the half-liter of milk.

Licorice will work, says Dr. Baschetti, only if the chronic fatigue sufferer also has enlarged and painful lymph nodes. "If you don't have these, you do not really have chronic fatigue syndrome," he says. Also, he insists that if you tend to have high blood pressure, you don't have chronic fatigue syndrome and certainly should not take licorice because it will cause sodium retention and raise blood pressure further, perhaps dangerously. Most important, licorice works only if you have low blood cortisol levels. This rules out people with depression (who may have been misdiagnosed with CFS), because recent studies show such depressed persons have high blood levels of the steroid corti-sol. Thus licorice in such cases would raise cortisol levels further, worsening the depression.

Important: Do not take licorice for chronic fatigue syndrome unless a doctor has diagnosed the condition. A correct diagnosis is absolutely essen-tial. Do not take licorice unless you have enlarged and painful lymph nodes. Do not take licorice if you have classic depression, unrelated to CFS. Do not take licorice if you have high blood pressure.

Fantastic
Blood Vessel Fixer

(GRAPE SEED OPC AND PYCNOGENOL)

It may cure many ills, but there's nothing like it for strengthening blood vessels and fighting varicose veins.

It's your lifeline—that intricate network of blood vessels, from tiny capillaries to large arteries and veins, that feeds blood to every bit of tissue from the top of your head to the tip of your toes. The integrity and strength of these blood vessels, combined with the proper functioning of your heart, are unquestionably paramount factors in your health and survival. If blood vessels grow old or diseased, fragile, thin, and leaky, your health is compromised. If blood-carrying oxygen doesn't flow through properly, your heart muscle can be damaged, your brain cells may die or malfunction, your leg muscles may cramp and cause pain, your vision may diminish. If a blood vessel leaks or bursts, you may suffer a brain hemorrhage or "bleeding stroke," or tiny spider veins may appear on the surface of your skin. Your gums and nose may bleed; varicose veins may bulge in your legs. Fluid may leak through permeable blood vessels, causing swelling or edema. Nothing is more critical than the vitality of those miles of capillaries, veins, and arteries that make up your circulatory system.

Yet has anyone ever told you of a medicine that can actually strengthen fragile and weakened blood vessels, restoring them to normal health, reversing and preventing circulatory disasters?

There is such a unique natural remedy—a drug extensively used in Europe with amazing success. There's no other medicine like it anywhere. Derived commercially from grape seeds and the bark of the pine tree, it is a mixture of antioxidant molecules, variously called proanthocyanidins, procyanidins, proanthocyanidolic oligomers (PCO), oligomeric procyanidins (OPC), pycnogenols (generic), Pycnogenol™ (pronounced pik-NOD-ja-nol), or just plain grape seed extract. And you can easily get it.

OPC, as it's commonly called in scientific circles, is expert at treating vascular diseases because it actually increases the structural strength of weakened blood vessels. It also has other biological activity and is one of the most potent antioxidants known—fifty times as powerful as vitamin E, according to some tests. Antioxidants can help neutralize the underlying chemical cause (free radicals) that promotes most diseases.

Research on OPC is just beginning in the United States, so there are few scientific data in American medical journals or textbooks to back up therapeutic claims. But there are four decades of proven use in Europe, especially France, to be excited about. Many Americans are already raving about the wondrous relief they have experienced from taking OPC, and its popularity is sure to soar as its benefits become even better known. Some experts call OPC a superstar among botanical supplements, the one with the most potential of all for benefiting human health.

What Is It?

In 1947 the renowned French chemist Jack Masquelier, professor emeritus of medicine at the University of Bordeaux, isolated the first OPC, a colorless substance, from the red skin of the peanut. He tells how he gave it to the wife of the dean of his faculty, who had severe edema from pregnancy; her swollen legs got so tired she could barely walk. "Well, the dean's wife was cured in forty-eight hours," says Dr. Masquelier. "So there had to be something special about my extract." In 1950 the peanut-skin OPC became the first vasculo-protective medicine, known as Resivit and sold in France. About a quarter of a century later another drug based on Dr. Masquelier's grape seed OPC, called Endotelon, made its debut in France. By 1979 Masquelier had also christened his brainchild "pycnogenols," a generic word describing in Greek its multifaceted chemistry. (Later the term Pycnogenol became a patented registered trademark of a British company, Horphag Research Limited.) Dr. Masquelier has also detected OPC in virtually all plants, red wine, and the peanut kernel itself. The current concentrated commercial sources are grape seeds and the bark of the French maritime pine tree. Dr. Masquelier also says OPC primarily accounts for the antioxidant, artery-protecting activity of red wine and tea.

What's the Evidence?

If you lived in France, you would probably know OPC best as a foremost drug to treat varicose veins, a potentially disfiguring, painful condition in which veins tend to sag and stretch, become inflamed, and appear as purplish, elongated bulges beneath the skin. Taking OPC, studies show, can actually strengthen the veins, firming them up and restoring their resilience so they retract back into the skin. Dr. Masquelier and colleagues have done nine studies confirming OPC's efficacy for varicose veins. Another primary use of OPC is to reduce fluid buildup, or edema. When vascular walls become weakened, fluids transported inside the veins leak out, leading to swelling. By strengthening capillary walls and performing other biological maneuvers, OPC reduces edema and swelling, which may be important in fighting high blood pressure, congestive heart failure, and sports injuries involving swelling. Additionally, OPC has been used to treat eye problems—glare, night blindness, macular degeneration—arthritis, hay fever and allergies, and nosebleeds.

"If you regularly take OPC, your vascular walls will be reinforced," says Dr. Masquelier. He cites ways to tell if you need OPC: "In the morning you brush your teeth and discover that your gums are bleeding. Or you notice a speck of blood on the cornea of the eye. Or at night you feel tired, your calves are swollen, you notice edema. In that case you're suffering from vascular fragility, and OPC fights all these pathological mechanisms."

DECADES OF EUROPEAN RESEARCH

Europeans for forty years have benefited from OPC treatment to relieve capillary and circulatory disorders, primarily varicose veins. And the research, much of it done by Dr. Masquelier and colleagues, is compelling. In 1995 a major review of the research by Italian investigators concluded that OPC indeed worked, sometimes better than other potent human-made pharmaceutical drugs. One 1981 well-conducted (double-blind) study of fifty patients with varicose veins found that 150 milligrams of grape seed OPC (Endotelon) a day worked faster and longer than a commonly prescribed pharmaceutical drug (Diosmine) in reducing pain, sensations of burning and tingling, and the degree of distention of the veins. All symptoms improved within thirty days. In another study, giving patients with widespread varicose veins just a single 150-milligram dose of OPC improved the tone of their veins, as meticulously measured by a standard test. Another 1985 double-blind controlled study of ninety-two French patients with "venous insufficiency," or varicose veins, showed that 300 milligrams of grape seed OPC daily for twenty-eight days reduced pain, tingling, night leg cramps, and swelling by more than 50 percent. Seventy-five percent of the patients improved on the grape seed medication, making it twice as effective as the dummy pill.

OPC has also proved good medicine for eyes. It helps eyes recover from the glare of bright lights, important in night vision. Two separate French studies of 100 subjects found that taking a 200-milligram dose of grape seed OPC for five weeks dramatically increased the recovery of visual acuity after being subjected to bright lights. In other tests the grape seed product also worked to relieve eye stress caused by working at a computer monitor and improved the function and sensitivity of the retina in nearsighted people. Several studies have found that OPC was successful in treating retinopathy that causes deteriorating eyesight, particularly in diabetics. The usual doses: 100 to 150 milligrams of OPC daily.

OPC's strong antioxidant activity may also make it ideal treatment for age-related macular degeneration, a serious eye disease, observes Dr. Denham Harman, antioxidant authority at the University of Nebraska. That's because OPCs "tend to localize in the small vasculature of the eyes," he says. Other weaker antioxidants have delayed progression of macular degeneration.

DR. DIXON'S MIRACLE
"It Stopped My Eye Disease"

Madison Dixon, age seventy-six, an optometrist in a small town in southern Georgia, had been using antioxidants, mainly vitamin C and beta-carotene, to retard two serious age-related eye problems— cataracts and macular degeneration—for nearly forty years. So when he heard about a new super- potent antioxidant from France called Pyc- nogenol, he was excited, thinking it might work even better to save sight. In particular he was wor- ried about the diminishing vision in his own right eye, due to macular degeneration, in which the macula, the tiny center of the retina, disintegrates, sometimes eventually causing blindness. There is no medical or surgical cure for the condition, although studies have shown that antioxidants can slow its progression.

Dr. Dixon started taking Pycnogenol in 1993. He was elated. His macular degeneration did not con- tinue to worsen, nor did his cataracts. "My vision uncorrected is still 20/30," he says. "I credit the slowdown of disease to first Pycnogenol and then grape seed extract." Initially he took eight capsules of Pycnogenol a day, dropping to two after four months. Then he switched to less expensive grape seed extract, which he finds just as effective for his eyes and even more therapeutic for his osteoarthri- tis. A big plus: The grape seed extract "costs about half as much."

Until his recent retirement he also recom- mended OPC grape seed extract and Pycnogenol to his patients, whose eyes, he says, invariably improved. "I do not know a single patient who did not benefit," he says.

The grape seed antioxidant performed another miracle for Dixon's wife, Jane, who has advanced rheumatoid arthritis, he says. She has had two knee replacements and one hip replacement, and was facing replacement of the other hip. "The doctor looked at an X-ray of the other hip and said, 'In about six months to a year we'll be doing that one,'" recalls Dixon. "That was about four years ago. The doctor is surprised, but we're not even thinking about surgery now. To tell the truth, since taking the grape seed extract, that hip gives her fewer problems than the one that was operated on."

DEFUSES HIGH BLOOD PRESSURE

OPC may help reverse high blood pressure and its consequences. People with high blood pressure commonly have weakened capillaries with high permeability, boosting their chances of hemorrhagic stroke and ruptured blood vessels in the retina of the eye, research shows. In animals prone to high blood pressure, OPC has strengthened capillaries, according to extensive studies by one of Hungary's most distinguished scientists, Dr. Miklos Gabor. In human terms this means OPC might keep blood vessels in the brain and eyes from weakening enough to burst, he says. Indeed, French researchers have found that grape seed OPC increased capillary resistance by 25 percent in patients with high blood pressure and/or diabetes, compared with those taking a placebo sugar pill. Exciting new research by Professor Peter Rohdewald, a leading pharmaceutical researcher at the University of Münster in Germany, shows that pine bark OPC reduces adrenaline stress reactions that trigger high blood pressure. In animals, brain damage from strokes was much less in those first given OPC.

In a particularly convincing demonstration of OPC's ability to increase capillary "resistance" or strength, Dr. Rohdewald and colleagues applied a vacuum to the skin of elderly people, which readily produced microbleedings within the skin. But after the subjects took a single dose of 100 milligrams of pine bark OPC (Pycnogenol), the vacuum power had to be increased markedly to produce the microbleeding. This means the OPC strengthened the capillaries so "they don't 'leak' or bleed as easily," said Professor Rohdewald.

Further, it is well known that inflammation and diabetes abnormally increase the permeability of blood vessels. Giving animals OPC blocked such detrimental increased permeability of brain capillaries, the aorta of the heart, and cardiac muscle capillaries, according to French scientists at the University of Paris.

MARIAN'S MIRACLE
"It Cured My Allergies"

European studies have also shown that OPC extracts suppress release of histamine. The implications are evident for those suffering from respiratory allergic reactions, notably hay fever. OPC can act as an antihistamine. Indeed, Marian Holtan-Jensen, director of new products at a major U.S. supplement company, was quite astonished to find that OPC stopped her pollen allergies of thirteen years after only three days. She had heard that OPC relieved allergies, but she didn't believe it. "I discounted it. I am a natural skeptic," she says. But when she was reviewing the scientific evidence for the French OPC drug Endotelon, now called Dr. Jack Masquelier's Tru-OPCs in this country, she saw research on its effectiveness as an antihistamine. She said, Well, okay, I'll try it. She had taken many antiallergy drugs, but hated them. "I took all kinds of prescriptions, such as Seldane, and everything I took left me feeling kind of dopey and semifunctional." She took the French-recommended 300 milligrams a day of Dr. Masquelier's OPC as an antihistamine. "Within three days, what had been a terrific case of blocked sinuses, runny eyes, and scratchy throat was gone. I was just amazed." She continues to take 150 milligrams of the OPC every day and has "never had another flare-up—even in the worst allergy seasons."

How Does It Work?

OPC's main claim to fame is its unique ability to strengthen the walls of blood vessels weakened by age and disease. OPC thus reverses the fragility of blood vessels, making them more intact and supple so blood flows through easily and doesn't leak out. OPC accomplishes this by actually creating tougher, thicker, more tightly knit blood vessel walls that are less apt to stretch, leak, or burst. As Dr. Masquelier explains, two proteins in the vessel wall, collagen and elastin, greatly determine the elasticity and permeability of the vascular wall, whether the wall is solid, strong, and flexible, or fragile and leaky. OPC attaches to these two building block proteins, preventing their degradation by destructive enzymes and encouraging their synthesis and maturation. In short, OPC reinforces the structure of the connective tissue that makes blood vessels strong and resistant.

Part of OPC's power in protecting blood vessels is its anti-inflammatory activity; inflammation is increasingly recognized as contributing greatly to the degradation of arteries and veins. OPC also acts as an antihistamine by blocking the activation of enzymes that regulate histamine release. "Although OPC was never released as a pharmaceutical antihistamine, it performs just as well," says Dr. Masquelier.

How Much Do You Need?
Recommended therapeutic doses of OPC are between 150 and 300 milligrams daily to treat illnesses and between 50 and 100 milligrams to maintain good vascular health.

The Safety Factor
OPCs are expected to be safe because they are widespread in the food supply; however, they have been tested for toxicity in laboratory mice, rats, guinea pigs, and dogs and have been declared nontoxic, nonmutagenic, noncarcinogenic, and free of side effects, according to a review of the evidence by German researcher Professor Peter Rohdewald. Additionally, in tests of OPC on humans, doctors have not reported adverse effects, say experts.

GRAPE SEED EXTRACT VERSUS PYCNOGENOL?
Commercially, you can get OPC as a grape seed extract or a pine bark extract (known as Pycnogenol, a brand name) or a combination of the two. There has been much controversy over which is better. It's well known which is less expensive—grape seed extract. Even the highest-quality grape seed extract is from one-third to one-half the cost of Pycnogenol. Moreover, nearly all the research in Europe

has been done on grape seed extract, mainly Dr. Masquelier's formula, not pine bark or Pycnogenol. Although new studies are now being done in both Europe and the United States using Pycnogenol, most of the claims for it actually stem from research on grape seed extract.

Thus the question among many practitioners is which to use and recommend. Seattle's Dr. Michael Murray, author of several books on the medicinal value of plant chemicals, argues that grape seed extract is generally superior to pine bark extract in proven efficacy and price. He points out that OPC from grape seed is recommended as the preferred form by health care practitioners in France, where it outsells Pycnogenol by 400 percent. The fact that Pycnogenol currently outsells grape seed extract in the United States, Dr. Murray says, is due to aggressive marketing and misinformation.

Consumer Concerns

The quality of OPC products varies greatly. And it's often impossible for consumers to know how much OPC most contain. Many reputable companies are now turning out grape seed extract with varying concentrations of OPC and other constituents. Yet standardized testing on OPC is rarely done to determine the amount, potency, and all-important bioavailability (how your body absorbs it). But there is good news for consumers about both pine bark and grape seed extracts. The Henkel Corporation, a well-respected U.S. supplement maker, has assumed marketing of Pycnogenol in this country (it is made in England) and is expected to upgrade the scientific testing and marketing of the supplement. However, Pycnogenol is still expected to cost much more than the highest-quality grape seed extract.

Also, you can now easily get Dr. Masquelier's original

French OPC remedy, which has been so thoroughly tested in Europe, notably as a treatment for varicose veins and other vascular diseases. The grape-seed pharmaceutical quality extract, known as Endotelon in Europe, is being sold by Nature's Way as Dr. Jack Masquelier's Tru-OPCs and by NaturaLife as Dr. Jack Masquelier's Authentic OPCs. Dr. Masquelier's brand name pine-bark OPC and a combination of grape seed and pine bark, known as OPC-85, which was found effective in recent research on attention deficit disorder, are also available through the company Primary Source by calling 800-667-1538.

Should You Try It?

If you think your blood vessels need help—undeniably blood vessels weaken with age and disease—taking OPC could be a smart idea, especially if you are older or concerned about varicose veins, spider veins, age-related deterioration in vision, swelling and edema, allergies, high blood pressure, a tendency to bleed and bruise easily, or a family or personal history of a bleeding stroke or diabetes (a disorder in which blood vessels are more permeable). There is no safe alternative, nothing comparable among other natural remedies, over-the-counter drugs, or even prescription drugs. OPC is safe and relatively inexpensive and could add a whole new dimension of health to a body with a poor and deteriorating circulatory system. Just think, if OPC reinforces the walls of any blood vessel, it does the same for all arteries, veins, and capillaries. It is not selective. The potential payoff is enormous in fighting vascular disease in all its destructive guises.

What Else Is It Good For?

Since OPC is an antioxidant, research shows it fights cholesterol by discouraging deposits from forming on artery walls. OPC's anti-inflammatory activity may help relieve inflammatory conditions, including arthritis, allergies, bronchitis, and asthma. OPC also corrects dangerous blood clotting tendencies that trigger heart attacks and strokes. Dr. Ronald Watson, a researcher at the University of Arizona, recently confirmed that OPC (Pycnogenol) normalizes platelet aggregation—blood stickiness leading to hazardous blood clots. He showed that when people smoked, their platelets clumped together in a tendency to form clots. But about twenty minutes after taking OPC, their platelets returned to normal.

IS IT ALSO BRAIN MEDICINE?

A surprising use of OPC has arisen among people suffering from that bewildering disorder in concentration and attention known as attention deficit disorder (ADD), or attention deficit with hyperactivity disorder (ADHD). It is said to have begun quite accidentally when people with ADD took OPC for another purpose, such as allergies, and noticed an improvement in concentration and mental focus, classic symptoms of attention deficit. Others started using it. Word spread, and the ADD remedy has achieved high visibility on the Internet and at natural products trade shows.

The use of OPC for this purpose has not been widely studied. But a preliminary study by Marion Sigurdson, Ph.D., a psychologist in Tulsa, Oklahoma, who specializes in treating attention deficit disorder, has found striking benefits from OPC. Using a blend of grape seed and pine bark (Dr. Masquelier's OPC–85 product), Dr. Sigurdson found that it worked just as well as the commonly prescribed stimulant medications, including Ritalin, on thirty children and adults diagnosed with ADD. The subjects were given a battery of computerized and behavior tests to judge their attention, concentration, and other important factors in ADD under various circumstances: when they were either on or off their usual stimulant medications, or on the OPC alone. When they wree off their medications, their ADD deteriorated. On their medications, they were much improved. But when they took daily doses of the OPC grape seed–pine bark mixture, their scores and behavior were just as improved as when they took stimulant drugs. In other words, the OPC equaled the drugs in most subjects. Generally, children fared better on a lower dose (20 milligrams of OPC per 20 pounds of body weight daily), and adults did better with a higher dose of 40 milligrams per 20 pounds of body weight daily. (Many of the subjects also had other positive effects: decreased heartbeat, disappearance of tennis elbow, relief of acne, improved sleep and mood.)

Scientifically, how could this possibly be true? How could mundane grape seed and pine bark chemicals have a profound influence on the brain comparable to that of a powerful pharmaceutical drug? According to Marcia Zimmerman, a California consultant who specializes in research on OPCs, there is some underpinning in the scientific literature, suggesting possible mechanisms of action. A fascinating way OPCs might affect brain cells, as shown by studies in cell cultures, she says, is by regulating enzymes that help control two crucial neurotransmitters—dopamine and norepinephrine, chemicals that carry messages among brain cells and are involved in "excitatory" responses. OPCs also help deliver nutrients to the brain, such as zinc, manganese, selenium, and copper, that are helpful in ADHD, according to recent research. Additionally OPCs' remarkable antioxidant activity may help stabilize brain cells and improve their functioning by neutralizing damage from free radicals.

STEVEN'S MIRACLE
"I Can Now Finish What I Start"

Looking back, clinical psychologist Steven Tenenbaum realizes he has always had problems concentrating, paying attention, and focusing. He did poorly in school, especially in math. "On my report card, it said 'Has no *Sitzfleisch'*—will not sit still," he recalls. He was hyperactive-impulsive and had problems with attention. But not until 1984, at age twenty-five when he was getting his doctorate at St. Louis's Washington University to become a psychologist, did he understand he had a neurological condition called attention deficit hyperactive disorder or ADHD, characterized by a short attention span, impulsivity, and sometimes hyperactivity. The condition is said to affect 4 to 7 percent of the population, both youngsters and adults.

Under ordinary circumstances, Dr. Tenenbaum would have relied on stimulant drugs, such as Ritalin, Dexedrine, or cylert, widely prescribed for ADHD. But he had learned to fly recreationally, and if he took such drugs he could not keep his pilot's license under Federal Aviation Administration (FAA) regulations. So he toughed it out for many years without medication. After getting his doctorate, he set up the Attention Deficit Center in St. Louis, which specializes in counseling and developing coping abilities in children with ADHD.

In 1995 he began to hear about alternative treatments for ADHD from patients, parents, and people on the Internet. The buzz on one such substance, Pycnogenol, was particularly fascinating to Tenenbaum. He tried it and was thrilled. "My effectiveness has increased by about 40 or 50 percent in the year and a half I've been on it. I can now finish what I start," he raves. Without his three-times-daily regimen of the pine bark extract, he becomes mentally scattered and unable to focus. "When that happens, I'll run to take the medicine (Pycnogenol), and fifteen minutes later I'll be calm, cool, and collected for about three and a half hours." He compares it to the stimulant drug cylert. "It functions like a stimulant in that it produces the increase in attention, the increase in focus, the decrease in emotional reactivity." He also feels it elevates his mood.

Tenenbaum notes that like prescription stimulants, the OPC seems to work for some but not others. It does not eliminate the problem, of course, but only helps control it. "It just dampens some of the intensity of the disorder," he asserts.

He is conducting a new study of Pycnogenol to treat ADHD, sponsored by the Henkel Corporation.

Potent
Cancer Therapy

(DIET AND SUPPLEMENTS)

It's the latest cancer treatment; the right stuff in
your diet can help control cancer, say patients
and doctors.

Could it be true that what you eat could help you survive cancer? In short, boost your chances of stopping
and even reversing cancer? For years many respected
authorities have scorned the idea. But as scientific evidence mounts, revealing a connection between diet and
chronic diseases including cancer, as well as the amazing
powers of antioxidants and other food constituents to
interfere with the cancer process, many experts are saying
yes, not only it could be true, but it probably is true. It's
no longer medically chic to denounce vegetarian and macrobiotic-type diets for cancer patients as "dangerous alternative nonsense." Plant-based diets as well as antioxidant
and botanical supplementation are becoming more
accepted in mainstream medicine, not necessarily as
magic bullets, but as a part of a multidimensional program that augments or "complements" conventional
surgery, radiation, and chemotherapy.

Indeed, using diet as cancer therapy is attracting some
prestigious mainstream attention. Pioneering Dr. Ernst

Wynder, president of the American Health Foundation in New York, has launched two major "nutritional intervention" cancer studies. In one five-year study of about 1,000 women, a low-fat (15 percent) diet is being tested to see if it thwarts recurrence of breast cancer. In the other, done cooperatively with New York's Memorial Sloan-Kettering Cancer Center, men with prostate cancer are put on a low-fat diet (high fat promotes prostate cancer) and given supplements of 800 IU of vitamin E, 200 micrograms of organic selenium, genistein (an antioxidant in soybeans), and soy protein. There's evidence all such supplements fight prostate cancer, says Dr. Wynder. The idea: to find out whether the diet and/or supplements curtail blood levels of PSA (prostate specific antigen), an indicator of prostate cancer activity. Dr. Wynder thinks everyone with cancer, especially breast, prostate, and colon cancers, should use dietary intervention as part of a comprehensive cancer therapy.

Thus, for an increasing number of doctors, it is no longer a heated contest of either conventional or "alternative" treatment alone, but a merging of the two to fashion the best course of treatment for the patient. And some cancer patients and even their doctors are calling the remissions they experience or witness miraculous.

JEAN'S MIRACLE
"All the Cancers Disappeared"

In August 1994, at age fifty-eight, real estate agent Jean Reinert went to a local clinic in Barrington, Illinois, a suburb of Chicago, for "a shot to clear up a cough." She had lost her voice from what she thought was a cold. The young doctor on duty became alarmed over two bumps at the base of her neck. He sent her for a chest X-ray. That night she got the shocking news: "large cell carcinoma of the left lung." Inoperable. Jean recalls an oncologist's death sentence: "It's starting to go up your windpipe and we are concerned that you are going to choke to death. The best we can do is buy you some time with radiation and chemotherapy." He gave her six months to live; she started radiation treatments.

By the end of September the cancer had invaded her brain. "After I started having trouble walking, they did a scan and found I had multiple tumors in my brain." Discouraged, but not willing to give up, she remembered having heard a speech by local physician Keith Block on treating cancer ten years earlier. She went to see him. "He was the first one to give me any hope." She recalls his looking at her X-rays and saying, "'These aren't very scary.' They were the nicest words I'd heard since I was first diagnosed."

In addition to her regular conventional therapy Jean started a "pretty strong nutritional program"—with supplements, "about forty of them, including vitamin C, coenzyme Q–10, bioflavonoids, garlic, and a "medically modified" macrobiotic diet, advised by Dr. Block. He also showed her how to do biofeedback, meditation, and positive imaging to further support her immune system. By December 1994 the news was quite astonishing. Scans showed the cancer mass in her lung was shrinking; the tumor was much smaller. However, to everybody's dismay, the cancer had spread to her spleen, descending aorta, adrenal glands, and bladder. She agreed to a five-month schedule of chemotherapy.

"Naturally, I was devastated to find out the cancer had spread so much," she remembers. But then she looked at it from the optimistic side. "I said, Well, I've almost gotten rid of my cancer in my lungs; I can get rid of the others, too." She intensified her efforts. "Every single day I imagined the doctor coming toward me smiling, saying, 'Your cancer is gone.' I would talk to God every day. I would call him big guy and say there are things I want to do I haven't done yet." She continued the nutritional program and the chemotherapy.

But in April 1995 they stopped the chemotherapy. There was no reason to continue. The scans could find no tumors to fight. All the cancers had disappeared. Her entire body was cancer-free. It remains so, at this writing, in February 1997. She still follows a "mostly macrobiotic" diet—grains, beans, vegetables, nuts, seeds, some fish, no meat, and very little sugar—and continues to take specific supplements recommended by Dr. Block.

NANCY'S MIRACLE
"They Thought I Was Already Dead"

The first place the cancer appeared was in her right breast. At age forty-seven, in 1989, Nancy Loewenberg had the breast surgically removed. But the cancer had already made its secret moves, invading her lymph nodes. It was quiet for five years. Then over the next year and a half, cancers showed up as a lump under her arm, tumors on her spine and hipbones, and a very large mass in her liver. She had radiation, more surgery, chemotherapy, but without success.

Throughout it all, Nancy says, "I never thought I was going to die." But the signs were grim. In June 1996, after radiation and three full courses of chemotherapy had failed, Nancy and her husband, Chuck, flew from their home in San Francisco to see Chicago physician Keith Block, whom they had read about. Dr. Block, as always, exuded optimism, but others feared Nancy was terminal. She arrived at Dr. Block's office in a wheelchair. "She was really so sick. Her bone marrow was suppressed from all the chemotherapy; she had little immune reserve," recalls Dr. Block. "When the radiologist saw the scans showing cancer throughout 75 percent of her liver, he actually thought I was showing him the scans of a person who had already died, because he didn't believe she could still be alive."

Nancy started treatment—chemotherapy with a different drug, nutritional supplements, a modified macrobiotic diet, body work, visualization—the comprehensive Block regimen as dictated by her particular biological profile. She remained in Chicago most of the summer and into the fall. Her response was evident fairly soon. After only two months, her blood markers of cancer activity on one test dropped from 12,000 to 135. The rapidity and extent of her response was surprising even to Dr. Block, who is no stranger to such events. By late September the cancers had virtually vanished. Scans showed she was nearly clear of all cancers in her bones and lymph glands, and only 3 percent of her liver remained cancerous. "All her cancer markers, which were quite abnormal before, returned to normal," says Dr. Block. "The radiologist, upon reading the new scans, was incredulous. He said 'This is miraculous' in exactly those words. It was a remarkable biological turnaround."

Nancy is now back in California and out of her wheelchair. She's on a new anticancer drug, a hormonal blockade, similar to tamoxifen. "Basically," says Dr. Block, "we are putting her on a long-term maintenance regimen. It's extraordinary what has happened to her. I wouldn't say we know what is going to happen to her in a year or five years down the road, because these are mean diseases and they frequently do show their faces again, but the point is she is relatively free of cancer now."

"I'm a miracle and I'm alive," says Nancy. But she knows the cancer might grow again. "I still have it with me." She does everything she learned at Dr. Block's "cancer spa," as she calls it, to keep it away. She eats a modified macrobiotic diet; she takes handfuls of antioxidants and other supplements, as well as the anticancer drugs. She credits all of them for her remarkable recovery, but she also credits her positive attitude. "Dr. Block says I shouldn't be worried, and I'm not."

What Is It?

An anticancer diet is mostly a vegetarian, natural foods, low-fat diet. It's well known that the Japanese have relatively low rates of certain cancers and, further, that even after cancer is diagnosed, its progression is often much less rapid than in Western populations. Why? Because the diet, rich in soybeans, vegetables, and fish, and lower in fat, slows down cancer growth, says Dr. Wynder. Not surprisingly, one of the most popular cancer diets—a macrobiotic diet—is derived from the traditional Japanese diet. It was popularized in this country by Michio Kushi, head of the Kushi Institute in Boston. Kushi's classic macrobiotic diet is meatless, low-fat, high-grain, high-vegetable. Prohibited or severely restricted: table salt, yeast, refined sugar, meat, dairy foods, eggs, poultry, tomatoes, most fats and oils, processed foods, and alcoholic beverages. Occasionally allowed: white fish, fruits, lightly roasted seeds and nuts. Percentage of fat is between 10 and 13 percent.

Such a rigid macrobiotic diet is difficult for Americans to adhere to and may not even be the best for some cancer patients; many doctors favor less restrictive "modified" macrobiotic diets. Also, in treating cancer, it's increasingly common to add antioxidant supplements.

What's the Evidence?

Evidence that eating fruits, vegetables, grains, and fish helps block the development of cancer is overwhelming. It's widely agreed that people who eat the most fruits and vegetables are only half as likely to get cancers of various types. Research also shows that certain foods and antioxidants arrest or slow down the progression and spread of cancer and increase survival times. Notable are broccoli, garlic, fish oil, high-fiber grains, soybeans, vitamin C, coenzyme Q–10, and selenium, as shown in clinical trials and practice, epidemiological (population) studies, or animal and laboratory cell culture tests. There's also abundant evidence that chemicals in meat promote cancer. Thus, it makes scientific sense that plant foods—the staples of an anticancer diet—could help curb cancer and that eating meat could encourage it.

Cancer is, after all, a longtime process, the manifestation of accumulated cell damage over decades, that continues to grow and metastasize, or spread. Interrupting the cancer process at any stage—including after a tumor is apparent—could help fight cancer. Many plant foods and constituents, as well as certain fats, kill cancer cells or block their spread in tissue cultures, increase survival from cancer in animals, or rev up immune functions and specific detoxification systems in the body that directly fight cancer. A few examples: Shiitake mushrooms contain lentinen that boosts immunity and inhibits growth of tumors. Garlic directly destroys cancer cells in petri dishes. Cabbage stimulates excretion in women of a type of estrogen that boosts breast cancer. Broccoli contains compounds that help rid the body of cancer-causing chemicals. Soybeans contain several chemicals, including genistein, that modify hormonal activity that promotes breast and prostate cancer. Fish oil revs up the body's natural antioxidant system. Harvard's George Blackburn finds that fish oil given to breast cancer patients before and after surgery tones down cancer activity and possible metastasis. Italian researchers find that fish oil blocks recurrence of colon cancer. Eating wheat bran cereal also has suppressed the growth of polyps that can lead to colon cancer, and the recurrence of the cancer after surgery.

Increasing evidence also finds that adding vitamins and minerals, particularly antioxidants, to conventional cancer therapy can make a dramatic difference. In an extraordinary display of cancer-fighting power, adding megadoses of vitamins, mainly antioxidants, to drug therapy for bladder cancer cut recurrence of the cancers in half and nearly doubled the survival time of patients, in a recent study. "The effects were dramatic," said researcher Donald Lamm, head of urology at West Virginia University in Morgantown. In his study of sixty-five patients, all took BCG, a standard immunotherapy drug. About half also got high doses of vitamins A, C, E, and B6. Over two years only 40 percent on the vitamins developed new tumors, compared with 80 percent taking the drug only. Vitamin takers' survival time was thirty-three months versus eighteen months for the drug-only group.

The cancer community is still agog over a spectacular 1996 study by Dr. Larry Clark of the University of Arizona, demonstrating the power of the trace mineral selenium against cancer. Taking 200 micrograms of selenium daily for about seven years reduced the occurrence of all cancers in a group of 1,300 older people by 42 percent and cancer deaths by nearly 50 percent compared with those on a sugar pill or placebo. Selenium had the greatest impact on prostate cancer, slashing occurrence by 69 percent. Selenium also decreased rates of colorectal cancer 64 percent and lung cancer 39 percent. It was an unprecedented cancer intervention study, and it bumped up the respectability of using supplements against cancer several notches.

Specific research also shows that a macrobiotic-type diet can fight cancer, according to Dr. John Weisburger, a noted cancer researcher, now at the American Health Foundation and formerly at the National Cancer Institute. After reviewing research, he concluded that such restricted plant-based diets can starve cancers, suppressing their growth. In particular, he cites a 1993 study by James P. Carter showing that patients with fairly advanced prostate or pancreatic cancer survived much longer than usual on a macrobiotic diet. Those who deviated from the diet "experienced tumor regrowth, occasionally with a fatal outcome," wrote Dr. Weisburger in the *Journal of the American College of Nutrition*. "The diet seemed to prevent tumor growth, but not cause tumor regression," he noted. It probably works by lessening intake of cancer promoters and increasing intake of cancer antagonists, Dr. Weisburger concluded.

Whether it is coincidence or not, a change in diet often goes along with spontaneous remission of cancers. In a study of cancer remissions in the Netherlands, Daan C. van Baalen and Marco J. de Vries of Erasmus University found in 1987 that dietary change was one of the factors most frequently associated with spontaneous regression of cancer.

It's never too late to use diet against cancer, as a preventive or a treatment. It should help at any stage.
—Dr. John Weisburger, cancer researcher, the American Health Foundation

HOW ONE PIONEERING DOCTOR DOES IT

One of the most respected pioneers of "complementary" cancer treatment is Keith Block, M.D., of Evanston, Illinois, the doctor who treated cancer patients Jean Reinert and Nancy Loewenberg. He is medical director of the Cancer Institute of Edgewater Medical Center in Chicago and a clinical instructor at the University of Illinois School of Medicine. Dr. Block designs an individual treatment regimen to fit each cancer patient, depending on the type of cancer and a complex analysis of the patient's own biochemistry. The treatment then encompasses options of conventional therapies, including surgery, chemotherapy, and radiation, plus a range of unconventional therapies, including nutrition, based on a macrobiotic, vegetarian, or fish-vegetarian diet, and supplements of vitamins, minerals, botanicals, whole foods, phytochemicals, and other agents with documented scientific validity. Nutrition is but one of seven components of his therapy. Foremost is conveying hope, giving the patient a positive attitude, a passion for life, the idea that "you can fight for your life." Next is proper medical care. "I believe in medical gradualism, starting with the least invasive, least toxic, least damaging approaches and incrementally moving up the ladder with more aggressive therapies as the need calls for. Of course, in some cases [such as Nancy's] I will go to the big guns right off." Also important: emotional interventions, such as cognitive therapy, meditation, hypnotherapy, prayer, biofeedback, whatever is appropriate.

His nutritional regimen is very systematic and detailed and varies slightly with each patient, depending on blood analysis. Essentially it's a macrobiotic diet without the dogma and restrictions. "If a man with prostate cancer wants to eat a tomato—forbidden on macrobiotic diets—I encourage it, because good research supports it." A recent Harvard study linked tomatoes to a lower risk of prostate cancer. Patients eat mainly cereals and grains, a wide selection of vegetables, legumes, soy products, fish, and natural sweeteners such as rice syrups. Considered especially detrimental to cancer patients is cancer-promoting meat and the omega–6 fat high in corn oil and most margarines. Such fats are on the "avoid" list. Okay are canola and olive oil in limited quantities. Overall fat intake is around 15 to 18 percent; a strict macrobiotic diet is 12 to 15 percent. Also, Dr. Block discourages consumption of dairy products, egg yolks, refined sugars, alcohol, and highly processed foods.

He has a list of recommended antioxidants, including vitamin C, vitamin E, and coenzyme Q-10. And he uses botanicals as warranted, such as echinacea, dong quai (a special Chinese herbal formula), and a concentrated mushroom powder that he developed, to stimulate immune functioning and increase the effectiveness of conventional drugs while diminishing their side effects.

To Block there's no question that lifestyle, which helps trigger cancer, also promotes its progression and recurrence. Thus changing diet and infusing the body with natural cancer-fighting compounds makes sense in recovering and remaining free of cancer. "Diet itself is not the answer to cancer," he says, "But I do believe that to ignore it, in light of the overwhelming research, is at best incomplete medicine."

The Safety Factor

For those with cancer, two major fears arise over nutritional cancer treatments in general. One concern: that patients will reject all conventional therapies, such as surgery, radiation, and drugs, that might help save their lives, to pursue a macrobiotic or other restricted diet as the only cancer treatment. This can delay legitimate and effective conventional therapies at a time early in the cancer when they are most valuable. Two, some macrobiotic-style diets are so restrictive that cancer patients become malnourished, actually decreasing rather than boosting their ability to fight off the cancer nutritionally. Too few calories, too little protein, too little of the right type of fat can strip the body of strength. There are reports of cancer patients dying of malnutrition from highly restrictive macrobiotic diets. A dose of common sense is required. Although some weight loss may be beneficial for cancer patients, wasting away or dipping below your "ideal" weight, which is usually what you were in your early twenties, can be extremely hazardous.

Should You Try It?

An anticancer diet makes sense, used in conjunction with other conventional treatments, as an adjunct therapy, not as a sole therapy. The same is true of megadoses of antioxidants and other vitamins and, for that matter, other natural substances. It's unlikely that one alone will act as a cure for cancer, but there's good evidence that many combined can support an individual's ability to survive cancer. Don't count on one or two magic bullets to fight cancer: It takes many streams to make a river, according to an old proverb.

The Great Undiscovered Pain Medicine

(PEPPERMINT OIL)

Why take an aspirin or Tylenol when a pleasant aromatic herb can get rid of your tension headache just as quickly?

If you often pop pills to stop the pain of tension headaches, you're hardly alone. But wouldn't it be better to cure your headache without resorting to such pills? A surprising, newly discovered natural remedy for common headaches does exist, but you won't see it on television commercials or on over-the-counter drug racks in pharmacies. In fact, this novel pain medicine remains largely undiscovered anywhere, except in Germany, where investigators have proved it very effective in relieving ordinary tension headaches, the type that torment virtually everyone occasionally.

Such stress-induced headaches are a curse of modern life, more prevalent in Western countries than the common cold. They are a source of widespread human misery and societal cost. Some suffering individuals pop an aspirin or Tylenol every day to get rid of tension headaches. We spend about $1 million on analgesics every year. Unfortunately we pay an even higher price for the extravagant use of these painkillers, because of their side effects. The quick relief of acute pain is a trade-off for more serious long-lasting health problems, such as bleeding ulcers and damage to the liver and other organs. Headache disorders cost the European Community an estimated 40 billion German marks yearly in medical care and lost work time.

In truth our use of pills may not be the most appropriate way to dampen headaches. Headache pain, after all, does not come from inside the brain; that organ feels no pain because it possesses no sensory nerves. Headache pain actually originates from tension in the outer linings of the brain, the scalp and its blood vessels and muscles. The pain may engulf the whole head or only the back of the neck, the forehead, or one side of the head, and can be mild or deep, sharp, and throbbing. Common tension headaches, say experts, are caused when the face, neck, and scalp tighten up, often because of stress. The pain can last for days or even weeks.

Since tension headaches originate in the outer surface of the head, perhaps cooling them down by applying something to the outside of the head might work. Say, peppermint oil? It may seem like an eccentric idea. But peppermint is an ancient medicine with soothing powers. And it can help relieve some of the ills of modern life. Indeed, new German research shows that rubbing peppermint oil on your forehead is just as apt to cure your tension headache as taking a Tylenol! Some experts say the minty oil can also be a "miracle cure" for some other ills aggravated by modern stress.

DONNA'S MIRACLE
"My Headache Goes Away Faster"

"It really is better than Tylenol, including Tylenol Extra Strength," says Donna Lewis, a speech pathologist at the William Beaumont Army Medical Center in Texas. She has used peppermint oil to cure tension headaches several times, after she learned the remedy was being used successfully in Germany. Depending on her level of stress, sometimes she gets headaches several times a month; sometimes she goes several months without one. "Usually the headache is focused over my right eyebrow, and a lot of times the pain extends all the way back to the middle part of my head." Typically she used to take at least two 500-milligram tablets of Tylenol Extra Strength. It usually worked, she says, but it takes "maybe forty-five minutes to an hour for the headache to go away, and sometimes it gets rid of the extreme pain but leaves a dull ache, and then I have to take another one to try to get rid of that."

Now Donna subdues the same "mean" headaches by putting peppermint oil on her forehead, and she likes it a lot better. In the first place, she thinks it works slightly faster than Tylenol, "under half an hour." Also, she likes the "cool sensation" on her skin and the "pleasant peppermint smell." And she feels better about not taking a pill. "Sometimes I feel like I almost OD on pain medication."

When she feels a tension headache coming on, she dips her finger in a special peppermint oil mixture and applies it "all across my forehead; sometimes I put a little more on the area where the pain is pounding."

The peppermint oil has worked well every time she has used it for headache. In fact, she told others in her office about it; several of them are also using it "with similar results." The peppermint oil Donna uses came from a health food store; she mixes it with pure grain alcohol that came from a bar. The mixture tends to separate, so she always shakes it up before putting it on her forehead. Otherwise, you don't get the wonderful cool sensation, she says.

After discovering peppermint, Donna has no intention of going back to Tylenol.

What Is It?

The leaves and flowers of the common peppermint plant contain a volatile oil that is 50 to 75 percent pure menthol. The oil is widely used as a food flavoring, but the plant has a long history as a medicinal. In ancient Rome, Plinius (Pliny) the Elder recommended applying peppermint leaves to the forehead to treat headaches. The ancient Egyptian Ebers Papyrus recommends peppermint to calm the stomach. For centuries Western and Eastern doctors have recommended peppermint as a digestive (carminative), an antispasmodic (inhibits muscle spasms), and a stomach soother.

What's the Evidence?

In Germany, where the therapeutic effects of peppermint oil are widely recognized, researchers were aware that peppermint oil and its main constituent, menthol, are reputed to have analgesic effects when put on the skin. In search of an alternative to headache drugs, they theorized that peppermint might work. After a series of preliminary studies, leading headache researchers at the Neurological Clinic at Christian-Albrechts University in Kiel, Germany, presented the first clinical proof in 1996 that peppermint oil applied to the forehead does reduce headache pain from tension headaches—just as well as a taking a standard dose of 1,000 milligrams of acetaminophen—better known as two tablets of Tylenol!

Dr. Hartmut Gobel and colleagues studied forty-one men and women ages eighteen to sixty-five who had suffered tension headaches—from one to twenty-two attacks every month—for two to forty years. The study was of rigorous design—a so-called randomized, placebo-controlled, double-blind crossover study. When a headache struck during the study, each participant used, as instructed, one of three possible remedies—either two capsules of acetaminophen, or a real 10 percent peppermint oil preparation, or a fake solution (placebo) with only a few drops of peppermint, which they spread across their foreheads. They repeated the peppermint oil application again fifteen minutes and a half-hour later. All the subjects used all the remedies at various times in attempts to cure their headaches. They also meticulously, using scientific criteria, recorded the course of each of their headaches for an hour. As astonishing as it may seem, in most subjects, regardless of gender, age, or duration and frequency of headaches, the peppermint oil was just as quick and effective at relieving the head pain as acetaminophen. Headache intensity began to diminish after fifteen minutes with both.

"We find that patients can benefit from peppermint oil no matter what their sex, age, and headache history," says Dr. Gobel. However, he notes a few people did not get relief, for unknown reasons. Generally, he says, peppermint oil appears "more effective for those with less frequent and shorter headache attacks." In some persons, taking Tylenol and using peppermint oil worked better than either alone, says Dr. Gobel. Nobody complained of any side effects from the peppermint therapy.

How Does It Work?

The main pharmacological agent in peppermint oil is menthol. Many tests show that menthol in peppermint oil relaxes smooth muscle. Research in animals shows that peppermint oil inhibits smooth muscle contractions, induced by two body chemicals, serotonin and substance P, that play large roles in regulating pain sensations. Peppermint also may relieve head pain by relaxing pericranial muscles that cover the skull. But the herb's muscle-relaxing powers are only part of the story in alleviating headaches, says German investigator Dr. Gobel. He speculates that peppermint oil interferes in headache pain transmission several other ways. It produces a long-lasting cooling sensation on the skin that may stimulate the skin's cold receptors, influencing pain transmission in the spinal cord. Peppermint also increases capillary blood flow, decreasing pain sensitivity in the skin.

HOW TO USE PEPPERMINT OIL
FOR TENSION HEADACHES
Here's advice from German researcher
Dr. Hartmut Gobel

- At the first sign of a tension headache attack, apply a light coating of the peppermint oil across the entire forehead from temple to temple and eyebrow to hairline. If you have occipital pain (pain at the back of your head), use it on your neck as well. Apply only enough oil so that the whole area is moist. It is not more effective to use more oil than adheres to the skin.

- You need not massage the oil into your skin; you can apply it with your fingertips or with Q-Tips or a small sponge of the type that comes with the German product.

- If the peppermint oil drips into your eyes, wash it out with water. It is not harmful but can cause a burning sensation in the eyes, or in any open wound.

- It is not necessary to wash your face before applying the oil. But the peppermint oil can remove or smudge makeup, which may need a touch-up after the oil has evaporated.

- Use peppermint oil only after a doctor has diagnosed tension headaches, especially if they are frequent, to be sure the headache is not due to an underlying organic cause that demands more serious attention and treatment.

PEPPERMINT OIL VS. SPASTIC COLON

One of the most perplexing, tormenting, and "incurable" modern disorders, causing pain and distress to millions of Americans, is called irritable bowel syndrome (IBS), or spastic colon. Its number one characteristic is intermittent abdominal pain—aching, crampy, burning, or sharp— with constipation, diarrhea, or both. There is no single test or routine treatment for the problem. It's a "functional" disorder, in which the intestinal tract doesn't contract normally. Just as hearts can beat abnormally, a condition called arrhythmia, the normal rhythmic contractions of the colon can also get out of whack and go into spasms. Nobody knows what causes it or how to correct it. It is one of the most disheartening conditions to try to treat, and doctors and patients often throw up their hands in despair. Interestingly, it occurs most often in high-stress people, who are also prone to tension headaches. (Irritable bowel syndrome is not to be confused with inflammatory bowel disease, quite a different condition.)

If peppermint oil can relax smooth muscle, maybe it could help fix the abnormal contractions of the colon. Doctors have long known peppermint has an effect in the GI tract. Peppermint's muscle-relaxing properties make it a culprit in heartburn. Peppermint tends to relax the sphincter muscle that separates the esophagus from the stomach. This allows an upsurge (reflux) of burning acid from the stomach into the esophagus. That's why experts tell people prone to heartburn to stay away from mints.

But more American doctors are now telling people with IBS or spastic colon to take peppermint oil. It may bring relief, according to scientific evidence. In Europe, notably the United Kingdom and Germany, peppermint oil is commonly used to relieve the symptoms of irritable bowel syndrome. Nearly twenty years ago studies appeared in British medical journals describing its successful use. Peppermint oil is officially endorsed by the German government's herbal remedies authority, known as Commission E, as an effective, safe treatment for irritable bowel syndrome. If you lived there, your doctor would surely offer you peppermint oil for spastic colon.

Many sufferers of the irritable bowel syndrome are told that it is a condition they will just have to live with. Before giving up hope, they should try enteric-coated peppermint oil.—Dr. Michael T. Murray, *Natural Alternatives to Over-the-Counter and Prescription Drugs*

Peppermint oil relieves the symptoms of spastic colon by relaxing intestinal smooth muscle, and British investigators have discovered why it happens. Peppermint acts as a calcium "antagonist" to block the influx of calcium into smooth muscle cells; calcium helps regulate muscle contractions. Thus peppermint appears to stop excessive muscle contractions and restore proper muscle tone in the intestinal tract.

The right kind of peppermint capsule—coated to resist stomach acid, so it is released in the small and large intestines—has relieved IBS, according to research in Great Britain and Germany. In one study sixteen patients with IBS got either enteric-coated peppermint oil capsules or a dummy pill for three weeks at a time. They rated their symptoms on a five-point scale, from excellent to terrible. The peppermint oil won out over the dummy pill. Subjects said it worked two to four times better than the placebo in relieving IBS. Only five on placebo said they felt better, compared with thirteen on the real stuff. Only one on the peppermint oil reported feeling worse.

Further proof that peppermint oil can block intestinal spasms comes from recent British research showing that the oil cut by 40 percent the incidence of spasms when it was put into the colon during a barium enema, according to a 1995 report in the leading British medical journal *The Lancet*. Researchers theorized that peppermint oil might also be a good thing to use during a colonoscopy (an internal examination of the colon) to prevent cramping up. The peppermint, they said, might be an inexpensive replacement for costly antispasmodic drugs now used to prevent spasms during such procedures.

How Much Do You Need?

For headache, use just enough peppermint oil to moisten the forehead. Apply it every fifteen minutes, or as needed.

The recommended dose of peppermint oil for spastic colon is one or two capsules daily of standardized enteric-coated peppermint oil capsules, each containing 0.2 milliliters of peppermint oil. Take them between meals.

The Safety Factor

In rare cases peppermint oil—applied to the skin or taken internally in capsules—has produced allergic reactions: skin rashes, rapid heartbeat, and muscle tremor. Heartburn is a possible side effect from internal use if you are vulnerable to the condition. The Food and Drug Administration classifies peppermint as generally regarded as safe (GRAS), used as a tea. Internal overdoses of peppermint oil in capsules could cause poisoning, characterized by mild respiratory distress, overexcitement, and, in extreme cases, convulsions. Pure menthol is toxic if ingested and can be fatal in small doses—as little as a teaspoon. Letting infants inhale menthol is extremely dangerous. Avoid using pure menthol.

Who Should Not Take It?

Don't give peppermint products to infants and very small children. Do not apply peppermint oil to the faces of infants or small children. Pregnant women should beware of ingesting peppermint products with high amounts of menthol because of the potential danger of miscarriage.

Consumer Concerns

The peppermint product used in Dr. Gobel's research was Euminz, made by Lichtwer Pharma in Berlin, and is widely advertised in Germany to treat tension headaches. It is not, at this writing, generally sold in this country. However, you can order it through the Merz Apothecary in Chicago, an old established pharmacy that specializes in German botanical medicines. It comes in a small bottle with a built-in applicator for convenience. The Apothecary's number is: 800–252–0275.

You can also mix your own peppermint solution. "It would be reasonably easy to do," says Purdue's Dr. Varro Tyler. Simply add one part (such as one teaspoon) of peppermint oil to nine parts (such as nine teaspoons) of pure grain alcohol, available at some liquor stores, and put it in a small bottle. Be sure to use the real peppermint plant oil, not one of the inferior mint plants, and do not add another oil, notably eucalyptus oil; it renders the peppermint oil ineffective. You can use a dab of cotton, a tissue, or your fingers to apply the peppermint oil to your forehead.

For spastic colon, use only an enteric-coated peppermint oil capsule, so it will pass through the stomach acid and into the lower intestine before disintegrating. Oil released in the stomach can cause heartburn. One enteric-coated brand, intended for the treatment of gastric symptoms associated with irritable bowel syndrome, is Colpermin, (Pharmascience, Inc., Montreal). Another is Peppermint Plus, made by Enzymatic Therapy in the United States.

Marvelous
New Heart Drugs

(VITAMINS C AND E)

They are the strongest, cheapest, safest heart medicine you can find. It's risky not to take them.

So your arteries are already narrowed or partially clogged from plaque buildup—nearly everybody's are to a degree by middle age, and more so as you get older. The artery walls are probably thickened and slightly stiff, no longer as flexible as when you were a child. The blood may not flow as smoothly through the openings as it once did. Maybe you have high cholesterol or high blood pressure, or you have already had a heart attack, a blood clot, a stroke, the chest pains of angina, or surgery to open an artery or even replace a heart. Maybe you are on cardiac drugs. In any event you, like most Americans, could probably use some safe new medications to help in overcoming the progressive disease known as atherosclerosis that afflicts more of us than any other disease.

You may not think of them as heart medicines, but they are. There's compelling new evidence that vitamin C and vitamin E can open up diseased and clogged arteries so they dilate normally and blood flows through to feed heart cells. These vitamins can also dramatically help slow down, stop, and maybe even reverse atherosclerosis, or "hardening of the arteries," by acting as anti-inflammatory agents and fighting bad cholesterol and other artery-clogging substances. They may even have a direct impact on heart function. In some research the vitamins proved more potent against heart disease than pharmaceutical drugs.

What makes all this so exciting is the fact that these vitamins can rescue us even after our arteries have become diseased and clogged. Thus we need not just sit around and do nothing, fearing the worst. The astonishing news is: If you can keep your arteries open, despite the amount of plaque buildup, you are not apt to suffer a heart attack. And that's one thing these vitamins can do, according to new findings and a new understanding of the role of artery function in heart attacks. They offer hope to millions who are not nearly ill enough to consider taking risky pharmaceutical heart drugs. They can also intervene in serious heart failure. That's why many doctors now say that antioxidant vitamins C and E in particular have crossed the line from preventive to therapeutic, becoming a new heart medication that can help save you from cardiac disability and death.

Some researchers and doctors are now pioneering the use of antioxidant vitamins as adjunct therapy to stop the deterioration of arteries and even to restore heart function and clear arteries, with amazing success. We are entering a new age of the practice of "antioxidant medicine," says Balz Frei, Ph.D., a prominent antioxidant researcher at Boston University Medical Center. In some cases heart patients are simply taking vitamin supplements on their own, sometimes with astonishing results.

JOEY'S MIRACLE
"Vitamins Opened Up My Blocked Arteries"

Joey Blackburn is by no means a typical case, but the remarkable reversal of her clogged arteries after she took a vitamin-nutrient supplement is intriguing.

In August 1990 Joey, age twenty, was diagnosed with viral cardiomyopathy, an uncommon type of heart disease in which a viral infection attacks the heart, often causing it to deteriorate into deadly malfunction. Doctors at St. Francis Hospital in Memphis, Tennessee, told Joey her only hope for survival was a heart transplant. Luckily a compatible heart was found, from an eleven-year old boy, and the surgery was performed in November 1990.

For five years Joey's annual heart catheterizations, or angiograms (X-ray pictures) that reveal the condition of her new heart's coronary arteries, looked fine. Then in January 1995 the news was "devastating." Her angiogram showed four serious blockages; all three main arteries of the heart were 90 percent blocked and a fourth vessel was about 60 percent closed. She had also gained nearly 100 pounds since her transplant, due partly to the immune-suppressant drugs, including prednisone, a steroid, and to overeating, she says. "My cardiologist, Dr. George Smith, was furious. He told me to go on a low-fat diet immediately." Frightened, Joey went on a strict diet. Four months later she was 30 pounds down, but still "so frustrated and so short of breath." She knew the restricted blood flow was slowly, steadily suffocating her heart. At the time she was not considered a suitable candidate for bypass surgery, a typical way to open coronary arteries.

Then a social worker on her transplant team at the hospital where Joey, a graduate of the University of Memphis, now works in medical records, suggested she try a particular type of vitamin amino-acid mixture, containing doses of vitamin C and other nutrients. Skeptical, Joey agreed, feeling she had nothing to lose. She started the vitamins in May 1995.

In November, six months later, she had a repeat catheterization. "My cardiologist could not believe it." Her cardiac catheterization report clearly documents a shrinkage of blockages in her coronary arteries. The 90 percent obstruction in the "left anterior descending artery" was now 70–80 percent; a 90 percent obstruction of the "second large diagonal branch proximal" had shrunk to 40–50 percent. A 90 percent obstruction of the "right coronary artery" had diminished to only a 40–50 percent narrowing. And the previous 60 percent obstruction of the "left circumflex coronary artery" was gone, and the artery appeared completely open.

Could the supplement account for the reduction of blockages in Joey's arteries? Judging from a description of the angiograms, Dr. Jay Johnson, a Nevada cardiologist and coauthor of an article in the *New England Journal of Medicine* on regression in coronary transplant disease, says, "It's possible." He agrees her case is "quite unusual, and it appears there was some regression," but he says there's no way to know because no studies on such vitamin use in transplant patients have been done. Also, if the vitamins did somehow partially reverse Joey's blockage, it probably involved effects on her immune system and not on factors, such as cholesterol and plaque buildup, thought responsible for ordinary heart disease, suggests Dr. Johnson. Nevertheless, such an event, although mysterious, may give new clues about how vitamins can work, and there is evidence that the same formula Joey used has worked to slow down the progression of atherosclerosis in people with ordinary coronary heart disease.

In early 1997 Joey did have bypass surgery to open an artery in her heart that became blocked for unknown reasons.

Consumer note: The formula used by Joey Blackburn is a patented combination of a nutritional supplement composed of vitamins, amino acids, minerals, and trace elements, developed by Dr. Matthias Rath. It is sold under the brand name Cellular Essentials Cardio-Basics, from Florida-based Rexall-Sundown International; and as Vitacor 20/90 from Health Now, Inc., a California-based research and development firm.

What Are They?

Vitamin C and vitamin E are potent antioxidants; this means they can block the destructive activity of chemicals in the body called oxygen free radicals. These free radicals are created internally by body metabolism and also enter the body through exposure to all kinds of chemicals, including air pollutants, cigarette smoke, fatty foods, and radiation. Free radicals attack cells, promoting malicious changes that underlie virtually every chronic disease. Free radicals are major culprits in heart disease; they promote buildup of plaque in arteries and abnormal vascular functions, such as dilation and contractions. Antioxidants block the deleterious activity of free radicals so they cannot destroy your arteries and heart.

What's the Evidence?

Evidence has been mounting over the last decade, showing that antioxidant vitamins, notably vitamins C and E, can ward off blockages of coronary arteries. Studies in monkeys, our closest relatives, have found that clogged arteries, induced by a high-fat diet, are prevented and reversed by modest doses of vitamin E. In a remarkable six-year research project Anthony J. Verlangieri, Ph.D., of the University of Mississippi's Atherosclerosis Research Laboratory, fed monkeys a high-fat lard-cholesterol diet. Naturally their arteries became clogged and blocked, but when the monkeys also got vitamin E, the extent of artery blockage dropped 60 to 80 percent. More spectacular, feeding the monkeys a daily dose of 108 international units (IU) of vitamin E *after* their arteries were seriously clogged cleared the artery blockage by about 60 percent. The blockages shrank from an average 35 percent artery closure to a 15 percent closure in two years!

Taking supplements of vitamins E and C also can retard artery clogging and open up arteries in humans. Dr. Howard N. Hodis at the University of Southern California School of Medicine found that men who said they took 100 IU or more of vitamin E daily after coronary bypass surgery had less narrowed arteries after two years than nonvitamin users or those taking lower doses of vitamin E. Furthermore, angiograms (X-rays) showed clearly that the plaque in the arteries of some of the vitamin E takers had shrunk, signifying a retreat or regression in atherosclerosis.

How dramatically vitamin E can be used to treat existing heart disease was revealed in a 1996 blockbuster study from the University of Cambridge in England. The study by Professor Morris Brown and Dr. Malcolm Michinson was conducted on 2,000 people with confirmed artery disease, including a history of heart attack. Over the next eighteen months, half the heart disease patients took a single daily dose of either 400 IU or 800 IU of natural vitamin E; the others took a placebo (dummy pill.) The results were so amazing that even the investigators were surprised. The users of either dose of vitamin E suffered only 23 percent as many nonfatal heart attacks as those taking the placebo. Vitamin E had slashed the incidence of heart attacks by an astounding 77 percent. The researchers pronounced vitamin E more powerful in controlling heart attacks than aspirin or cholesterol-lowering drugs. Indeed, they found that vitamin E reduced the risk of nonfatal heart attack to normal—that expected in healthy individuals with no signs of heart disease. Further, the benefits of the vitamin-drug were evident within six and a half months after subjects started to take it.

THE VITAMIN C MIRACLE

Vitamin C, long overshadowed by vitamin E as a heart protector, is now emerging as a prime-time superstar. The use of vitamin C as a heart disease treatment is one of the hottest new subjects of research. Exciting new studies find that vitamin C has a fascinating, newly discovered role in keeping arteries open. In the last few years scientists have established that artery clogging due to cholesterol and buildup of plaque, which vitamin E superbly discourages, is but one factor in triggering heart attacks and heart failure. Critically important also is so-called vascular function—how the cells lining the walls of arteries relax and contract.

"It's well known that people with coronary artery disease and diabetes have impaired vascular function," explains prominent antioxidant researcher Dr. Balz Frei at Boston University. This means their arteries do not relax enough to create a proper opening to accommodate blood flow. In normal individuals an artery may dilate about 15 percent during a common test. In heart disease patients the dilation is typically only 2 to 3 percent. This inability of arteries to relax normally is a major factor in heart attacks, says Dr. Frei. Here's why: If the artery fails to widen, for example, at the same time a small clot forms on an artery wall, blood flow may be blocked, starving and damaging heart muscle—in other words, creating a heart attack. But if arteries stay relaxed, even though they are narrowed by a clot and plaque buildup, blood has a much better chance of flowing through, so a heart attack doesn't happen. Abnormal vascular function is also what causes arteries to constrict, bringing on angina or chest pain, says Dr. Frei.

Now what if there was a drug to overcome abnormal vascular function that puts millions of Americans in jeopardy? There is. It is vitamin C. New research shows vitamin C can quickly correct abnormalities in the vascular functioning of diseased arteries that lead to heart attacks and angina.

In one recent test of forty-six patients with coronary heart disease documented by angiogram, Dr. Frei and colleagues Joseph A. Vita and John Keaney, Jr., reversed the dysfunctional way arteries relaxed by giving patients a dose of 2,000 milligrams of vitamin C. Ultrasound clearly showed that two hours after taking vitamin C, dilation of an artery in the arm improved by 50 percent in most patients and even more in those with the greatest initial vascular dysfunction. Indeed, after they took vitamin C the vascular function of the arteries in patients with heart disease was perfectly normal, dramatically reducing chances that the artery would malfunction, triggering a heart attack. Vitamin C, the researchers suggest, works primarily as an antioxidant to zap free radicals that otherwise suppress activity of nitric oxide needed to keep arteries properly relaxed. New studies are under way using 500 milligrams of vitamin C daily for heart patients for a month to see if the lower dose preserves normal artery function over a longer period of time.

Harvard researchers have shown that infusing vitamin C directly in the arteries of the heart also corrects vascular impairment in diabetics, which is similar to that in heart patients.

Another fascinating study showing that vitamin C and possibly vitamin E maintain good vascular functioning, even in the face of a high-fat diet, was done by researchers at the University of Maryland. Twenty faculty members, supervised by cardiologist Gary Plotnik, each ate a 50 percent fat, 900-calorie breakfast at McDonald's, consisting of one Egg McMuffin, one Sausage McMuffin, and two servings of hash browns. Using ultrasound, the researchers scanned the main artery of their arms. As expected, the fat burden caused their arteries to dilate abnormally, so blood flow was sluggish.

On another day the same subjects ate the same breakfast, except that this time, about fifteen minutes before pigging out, they took 1,000 milligrams of vitamin C and 800 IU of vitamin E. The results were astounding. The ultrasound showed that despite the fat overload, the subjects' arteries continued to dilate normally, allowing a normal blood flow to feed the heart muscle. Indeed, the vitamin C reversed a major ill effect of the high-fat breakfast that otherwise could trigger heart attack. The benefits lasted for six hours. This confirms the mounting evidence that vitamin C is a potent medicine for regulating artery functions.

THE JAPANESE MIRACLE

In another landmark study vitamin C was successfully used as a postangioplasty drug to keep arteries open, according to Japanese cardiologists at the Tokai University in Kanagawa. Angioplasty is a procedure often used to unblock clogged arteries. Because the arteries frequently close up again within several months, doctors are always looking for ways to prevent this reclosure. In the new Japanese study of 119 patients a daily dose of 500 milligrams of vitamin C was incredibly effective. Four months after the surgery only 24 percent of those who took vitamin C had reclosed arteries—or restenosis, as it is called—compared with 43 percent of the patients who did not get vitamin C.

By anybody's standards it was a blockbuster result. A modest dose of an absolutely safe pill costing a few cents a day nearly *doubled* the chances of a successful heart procedure. Further, it reduced the need for repeat surgery by about 60 percent. Only 12 percent of those who took vitamin C needed another heart procedure, compared with 29 percent of those who were not getting vitamin C. Harvard professor Thomas Graboys, director of the Lown Cardiovascular Center at Brigham and Women's Hospital in Boston, agrees that vitamin C "can't hurt and may help" in treating people with heart disease.

CHOLESTEROL BUSTER

Taking vitamin C can also lower bad LDL cholesterol, according to a well-designed (double-blind randomized) study in Australia. Taking 1,000 milligrams of vitamin C depressed LDL cholesterol by 16 percent after four weeks. A gram of vitamin C can also lower blood pressure, according to U.S. Department of Agriculture studies. Among people with high blood pressure a daily 1,000-milligram dose of vitamin C reduced both systolic (upper number) and diastolic (lower number) pressure about 7 percent.

How Does It Work?

The main way vitamin E fights heart disease is probably by its profound effects on blood cholesterol. It does not necessarily lower cholesterol, but it helps stop bad LDL cholesterol from being chemically changed (oxidized or turned rancid), a process that promotes cholesterol's ability to infiltrate artery walls, creating destructive plaque. Studies in animals and humans consistently show that a daily dose of 400 to 500 IU of vitamin E drastically inhibits the propensity of LDL to become toxic and damage arteries. Studies show that vitamin E also can slow down the proliferation of smooth muscle cells that pile up on artery walls, contributing to artery-clogging plaque.

Vitamin C, acting as an antioxidant, also protects arteries by neutralizing bad LDL cholesterol, but, as mentioned previously, vitamin C is a powerful vasodilator, and that is probably its more important method of fighting heart disease.

Actually vitamin C is a miracle drug mainly because it activates or releases the chemical nitric oxide in artery walls. Nitric oxide, according to a rush of new research, is an amazing chemical. It controls the relaxation and constriction of arteries that maintain or cut off blood flow to the heart and brain. Moreover, nitric oxide inhibits the proliferation of smooth muscle cells that accumulate to build up the mass known as atherosclerotic plaque. Thus, indirectly through manipulating nitric oxide, vitamin C influences artery health. However, vitamin C does even more. Blood clots tend to form on artery walls where a bit of plaque ruptures because it is weak and unstable. Scientists now realize that it is not primarily the *amount* of plaque lining your artery walls that creates heart attacks, but the *stability* of the plaque. If the composition of the plaque is stronger and less apt to rupture, clots and heart attacks are less apt to ensue. And what makes plaque more stable? Vitamin C, by spurring production and repair of collagen, a kind of cement that keeps plaque from fragmenting and creating hazardous blood clots.

How Much Do You Need?

Generally research shows that you need from 500 to 1,000 milligrams of vitamin C daily and from 400 to 800 IU of vitamin E daily to have a pharmacological effect on arteries and the heart.

The Safety Factor

Vitamins E and C are some of the safest substances known, even in high doses, far more than the doses needed for therapeutic effects. Vitamin C does not cause kidney stones, as once believed, or other significant side effects. There is no long-term toxicity for either vitamin. Vitamin E can have a slight blood thinning effect; check with your doctor if you are taking other heart medications, especially anticoagulants. Generally authorities do not advise taking more than 1,000 IU of vitamin E daily, except on the advice of a doctor.

Consumer Concerns

California researchers have found that synthetic vitamin E (dl-alpha tocopherol) protects LDL cholesterol from oxidation as well as slightly more expensive natural vitamin E (d-alpha tocopherol). However, many antioxidant experts favor natural vitamin E, and that form was used in the highly successful Cambridge study. Vitamin C of any type appears to work. The type effective in Dr. Frei's artery study was a low-cost brand from a drugstore. Reports that a more expensive vitamin C called Ester-C is superior have not held up. In fact, one study found plain old vitamin C better as an antioxidant.

What Else Are They Good For?

Antioxidant vitamins, including vitamins E and C, are being tested and used to treat a number of diseases—cancer, asthma, infertility, diabetes, arthritis, degenerative eye diseases, and degenerative brain diseases, such as Parkinson's and Alzheimer's. If you have asthma, for example, you might try a daily dose of 1,000 to 2,000 milligrams of vitamin C. According to a new analysis there have been eleven studies of the treatment of asthma with vitamin C since 1973. Fully seven studies found improved breathing in vitamin C takers. Taking 1,000 milligrams of vitamin C daily has reversed infertility in some males.

High doses of vitamin E (1,000 IU daily) normalized blood sugar in diabetics. Combinations of antioxidants, including vitamin E and C, have slowed the progression of cataracts and macular degeneration, a serious age-related eye disease sometimes resulting in blindness.

CONSUMER INFORMATION
AND ADVICE

ADVICE ON BUYING AND USING NATURAL REMEDIES

Obviously the more you know about natural remedies, in particular ones you are interested in using, the better. And the more serious the disease you are attempting to treat, the more care you must exercise and the more you must know. There is no substitute for knowledge, as the doctors, scientists, and patients cited in this book will tell you.

If there is one thing to keep uppermost in your mind, it is that many natural remedies, particularly those that have effects on serious diseases, such as congestive heart failure, depression, cancer, and chronic fatigue syndrome, must be approached with respect. They work because they have strong pharmacological activity. Although their side effects are generally much less than those of prescription pharmaceuticals—which makes them especially attractive—natural remedies if abused or overused can also harm you.

In the best of all worlds, you would have a highly trained person—a pharmacist, a doctor, or another health professional—to help guide you: to tell you what you need, how to decide among products and brands, how much to take, what to expect—just as you do when you buy prescription drugs. That's the situation in Germany, where both physicians and pharmacists must be knowledgeable about natural remedies, their approved uses, their potential side effects, and how they should be prescribed. In this country, where natural remedies are virtually ignored by medical schools and poorly regulated by the government, there is no nationwide established repository of consumer information or support system. That is sure to change in the near future, as the power of natural medicines becomes more known. However, at the moment, you are on your own.

In the various chapters of this book you have read advice about specific natural remedies. Here is some more general advice that may help you in your quest to use these marvelous medicines.

Talk to Your Doctor

Engage the support of your primary health care practitioner, if possible. Health professionals can keep you from making a major mistake. There are limits to self-diagnosis and self-care. You need to be sure in the first place that the disease you believe you have is in fact the disease you have. Professionals can save you from treating something that does not exist or failing to treat something that does. If the remedy doesn't fit the disease, of course it won't work, and you could be neglecting to recognize and treat a serious or life-threatening disease.

Further, health practitioners can help you gauge the extent of your success. Although just feeling better is a good indication that a natural remedy is working, it's best to have concrete evidence that can be provided only by health professionals. Sophisticated tests are often necessary to measure your true progress—for example, in judging changes, such as liver function tests when you are using milk thistle. Health professionals can help you integrate the natural remedies into your overall treatment. Remember, a natural medicine, notably in the case of cancer, should be part of a comprehensive treatment. Well-trained professionals can give you excellent advice on potential interactions with other drugs you may be taking. And of course they are essential if you get into any type of trouble while taking a natural remedy.

For most Americans a health practitioner means a doctor, usually a medical doctor—an M.D. You are lucky if you have or can find a doctor who is attuned to the use of natural remedies. And, happily, more physicians than ever before are becoming aware of the potential of natural remedies and integrating them into their practices. Some doctors say they learn much from their patients on this subject. Approaching your physician about a natural remedy you want to use is a good idea and essential if you have a serious illness. If your doctor is not responsive, you may want to seek help elsewhere.

For some Americans another very good possibility is a licensed or well trained naturopathic doctor, or N.D. Of all health professionals in this country, these are the best educated and trained in the use of natural remedies. Unfortunately they are in short supply—and concentrated in the northwest part of the United States. But as of early 1997 they were licensed as medical practitioners in twelve states: Alaska, Arizona, Connecticut, Florida, Hawaii, Maine, Montana, New Hampshire, Oregon, Utah, Vermont, and Washington. They are also licensed in four Canadian provinces: British Columbia, Manitoba, Ontario, and Saskatchewan.

Some well-trained N.D.s may be good practitioners but still unlicensed simply because their state simply doesn't offer licenses. Some unlicensed people, however, might call themselves naturopaths even though their training is from brief correspondence courses.

When choosing a naturopathic doctor the main question to ask is: Where did you graduate from? To be considered for a license N.D.s must graduate from an accredited naturopathic medical school, pass board-certified exams, and receive continuing medical education. At the beginning of 1997 there were two accredited schools: Bastyr University in Seattle and the National College of Naturopathic Medicine in Portland, Oregon. In addition, two schools were candidates for accreditation: Southwest College of Naturopathic Medicine and Health Sciences in Tempe, Arizona, and the Canadian College of Naturopathic Medicine in Toronto, Canada.

Licensed N.D.s can legally diagnose and treat illness, and can order diagnostic tests, including blood tests, X-rays, and ultrasounds. If you live in an area that licenses naturopaths you can use an N.D. as your primary care doctor, as well as an M.D. Otherwise only an M.D. can legally diagnose and treat disease. An N.D. often offers nutritional counseling or a nonprescription alternative for a chronic condition. In the case of a serious illness, such as cancer, naturopaths are trained to make referrals to M.D. specialists for conventional treatment.

How to Get the Best Products
Sometimes walking into a health food store or perusing the mail order catalogues for natural remedies is a nightmare of confusion, even for highly sophisticated, knowledgeable people. The array of different products and brands is daunting.

Since the government does not regulate the potency of natural remedies, you have no guarantee that a product you buy has substantial pharmacological activity. Sadly, some unscrupulous manufacturers market natural remedies that, when analyzed, have few or no active constituents.

Throughout this book you will find mention of certain outstanding brands of specific natural remedies. Here are some other ways to be sure you get good, efficacious, safe products.

- BUY FROM A GOOD COMPANY
  Since the industry is unregulated, your best bet is to choose products made by large, reputable companies that have been in business a long time and have a lot to lose by putting out a shoddy or deceptive product. Many of the excellent products increasingly found on American shelves originate in foreign countries, notably Germany and France, and are essentially the exact high-grade medicinal product used there and sold under a different name in the United States. For example, Ginkgold (ginkgo biloba) and Thysilin (milk thistle) are both made by large German companies. Because such remedies must meet the strict standards of Germany, they inspire confidence. Many large European companies, such as Indena in Italy, are now formulating their successful high-quality botanical remedies for an American market. If in doubt, ask your pharmacist or personnel in your health food store to direct you to well established supplement companies with excellent regulations for producing quality products.

- CHECK THE LABEL
  Your best guarantee of potency is to look for the word "standardized" on the label. This tells you that the product consistently contains a certain percentage of a specific chemical, which, in most cases, has been shown to be or is suspected to be the most active pharmacological agent. Because the manufacture of such products is more rigorous, they are usually more expensive, but generally worth it.

- CONSIDER THE PRODUCT'S FORM

An extract, which is either liquid, powder, or solid, is generally best. Such extracts are made by processing an herb in water, alcohol, or other solvents, in a way that isolates and concentrates its active constituents. Thus you can tell how much of certain agents a product contains. Bulk herbs can lose their potency quickly, and dried herbs stuffed into capsules are often worthless.

- CHOOSE SINGLE-INGREDIENT REMEDIES

As a general rule, beware the "kitchen sink" combinations. Some manufacturers combine mixtures of herbs that sometimes have little logic and serve to drive up the price or create a unique product of dubious value. If you want echinacea, buy it alone; the fact that it may be combined with goldenseal or another herb does not necessarily make it better or more potent. The same goes for other products. If you need ginkgo to boost your memory, it's better to get it full strength than to get a product diluted with ginseng, garlic, and other herbs.

- WHAT ABOUT PRICE?

Unfortunately cheapest is not always best. It's true some natural products are overpriced for various reasons. But in the realm of botanical medicines, the higher price often reflects higher quality. This issue is not as critical for vitamins. A less expensive vitamin C is apt to be as potent as a more expensive one, for example, although slightly higher-priced vitamin C tablets are often more pleasant and easier to swallow.

TEN THINGS YOU MUST CONSIDER:
TIPS FOR BUYING AND USING NATURAL REMEDIES

1. Don't take natural remedies for serious diseases that you have self-diagnosed.
2. If you are taking prescription medications, don't substitute or add natural remedies without first consulting your doctor or other health professional. A sudden cessation of medication and/or a drug interaction with natural remedies could be hazardous.
3. Buy extracts, liquid, solid, or powdered remedies when possible; they best preserve the potency of the herb's active constituents. Tinctures and freeze-dried encapsulated herbs are okay, too.
4. Buy a "standardized" product, as noted on the label, when possible. This means the product contains a certain percentage of one or more of the herb's reputed active compounds. "Standardized" products are usually more expensive.
5. If possible, buy from a top-quality company, which is usually a large, established manufacturer.
6. Don't take higher doses than the label recommends.
7. Generally buy single-substance products instead of formulas of mixtures of herbs or natural chemicals.
8. If you have any unusual symptoms—such as allergies, rashes, or headaches—after taking a natural remedy, stop taking it immediately and see a doctor if symptoms persist or are serious.
9. If possible take natural remedies with the supervision of a health professional who can monitor your progress.

10. If you are pregnant or nursing an infant, or have a chronic or serious health problem, check with your doctor before taking natural remedies.

WHERE TO GET ADDITIONAL INFORMATION

Organizations

American Botanical Council
P.O. Box 201660
Austin, TX 78720
Fax: 512-351-1924
E mail: custserv@herbalgram.org
web: www.herbalgram.org

The nation's leading source of reliable information on herbal remedies, including:

- The German Commission E Monographs, the American Botanical Council's English translation of 410 monographs on 324 herbs used in Germany with recommended dosages, approved uses, contraindications, and side effects. $189
- A professional quarterly magazine, HerbalGram
- A 32-page 4-color Education catalog listing more than 300 books: $2.50

American Herbalist Guild
c/o Planetary Formulas
Box 533
Soquel, CA 95073

American Herbal Products Association
P.O. Box 30585
Bethesda, MD 20824-0585

Herb Research Foundation
1007 Pearl Street
Suite 200
Boulder, CO 80302

Books
Bloomfield, Harold H. *Hypericum and Depression*. Los Angeles: Prelude Press, 1996.
Brown, Donald J. *Herbal Prescriptions for Better Health*. Rocklin, Calif.: Prima Publishing, 1996.
Bucci, Luke. *Pain Free: The Definitive Guide to Healing Arthritis, Low-Back Pain, and Sports Injuries Through Nutrition and Supplements*. Fort Worth, Tex.: Summit Group, 1995.
Castleman, Michael. *The Healing Herbs: The Ultimate Guide to the Curative Power of Nature's Medicines*. Emmaus, Pa.: Rodale Press, 1991
Duke, James A. *The Green Pharmacy*. Emmaus, Pa.: Rodale Press, 1997
Fugh-Berman, Adriane. *Alternative Medicine: What Works*. Tucson, Ariz.: Odonian Press, 1996.
Gordon, James S. *Manifesto for a New Medicine*. Reading, Mass.: Addison-Wesley Publishing Company, 1996.
Murray, Michael T. *Encyclopedia of Nutritional Supplements*. Rocklin, Calif.: Prima Publishing, 1996.
Murray, Michael T. *Natural Alternatives to Over-the-Counter and Prescription Drugs*. New York: William Morrow and Company, 1994.
Murray, Michael T. *The Healing Power of Herbs*. Rocklin, Calif.: Prima Publishing, 1991.
Pizzorno, Joseph. *Total Wellness*. Rocklin, Calif.: Prima Publishing, 1996.
Passwater, Richard, and Chithan Kandaswami. *Pyc-*

nogenol: The Super "Protector" Nutrient. New Canaan, Conn.: Keats Publishing, 1994

Sahelian, Ray. *Melatonin: Nature's Sleeping Pill*. Marina Del Rey, Calif.: Be Happier Press, 1995.

Sinatra, Stephen T. *Optimum Health*. Gatlinburg, Tenn.: Lincoln-Bradley Publishing Group, 1996. Also available in paperback. New York: Bantam Books, 1997.

Theodosakis, Jason, Brenda Adderly, and Barry Fox. *The Arthritis Cure*. New York: St. Martin's Press, 1997.

Tyler, Varro E. *Herbs of Choice*. Binghamton, N.Y.: Hawthorne Press, 1994.

———. *The Honest Herbal*, 3rd ed. Binghamton, N.Y.: Hawthorne Press, 1993.

Weil, Andrew. *Spontaneous Healing*. New York: Alfred A. Knopf, 1995.

SELECTED REFERENCES

Much of the material in this book comes from personal interviews with researchers, patients, and authorities on a specific topic, both in the United States and other countries, for which, obviously, there are no published references. Additionally, here are some of the most important published reports on specific remedies in the scientific literature. The articles can be found primarily in medical libraries. Only names of first authors are listed.

CANCER DIET THERAPY

Birt, D. F. Diet intervention for modifying cancer risk. Prog Clin Biol Res 395:223–34, 1996.

Block, G. Vitamin C and cancer prevention: the epidemiologic evidence. American Journal of Clinical Nutrition (Suppl) 53: 270S–282S, 1991

Carter, J. P. Hypothesis: dietary management may improve survival from nutritionally linked cancers based on analysis of representative cases. Journal of the American College of Nutrition 12(3): 209–226, 1993.

Clark, L. C. Effects of selenium supplementation for cancer prevention in patients with carcinoma of the skin. A randomized controlled trial. Journal of the American Medical Association 276 (24): 1957–63, 1996.

DeCosse, J. J. Effect of wheat fiber and vitamins C and E on rectal polyps in patients with familiar adenomatous polyposis. Journal of the National Cancer Institute 81(17): 1290–1297, 1989.

Goodman, M. T. Dietary factors in lung cancer prognosis. European Journal of Cancer 28 (2/3): 495–501, 1992.

Steinmetz, K. A. Vegetables, fruit and cancer prevention: a review. Journal of the American Dietetic Association 96 (10): 1027–39, 1996.

———. Vegetables, fruit and colon cancer in the Iowa Women's Health Study. American Journal of Epidemiology 139(1): 1–15, 1994.

van Baalen, D. C. Psycho-Social correlates of Spontaneous regression in Cancer. Monograph, Department of General Pathology. Medical Faculty, Erasmus U., Rotterdam , the Netherlands. April 6, 1987.

Weisburger, J. Guest editorial: a new nutritional approach in cancer therapy in light of mechanistic understanding of cancer causation and development. Journal of the American College of Nutrition 12(3): 205–208, 1993.

Zhang, Y. A major inducer of anticarcinogenic protective enzymes from broccoli: isolation and elucidation of structure. Proceedings of the National Academy of Sciences 89: 2399–2403, 1992.

ECHINACEA

Braunig, B. Echinacea purpurea radix for strengthening the immune response in flu-like infections. Zeitschrift Phytother 13: 7–13, 1992.

Melchart, D. Immunomodulation with echinacea—a systematic review of controlled clinical trials. Phytomedicine, vol. 1: 245–254, 1994.

Schoneberger, D. The influence of immune stimulating effects of pressed juice from Echinacea purpurea on the course and severity of colds. Forum Immunologie 8: 2–12, 1992.

Wagner, H. Immunostimulatory Drugs of Fungi and
Higher Plants. Economic and Medicinal Plant
Research 1: 113–45, 1985.

FEVERFEW

Johnson, E. S. Efficacy of feverfew as prophylactic treatment of migraine. British Medical Journal 291:
569–73, 1985.
Murphy, J. J. Randomized double blind placebo controlled
trial of feverfew in migraine prevention. Lancet 2:
189–192, 1988.

OMEGA–3 FISH OIL

Belluzi, A. Effect of an enteric coated fish oil preparation
on relapses in Crohn's disease. New England Journal
of Medicine 334: 1557–1616, 1996.
Billman, G. E. Prevention of ischemia-induced ventricular
fibrillation by omega–3 fatty acids. Proceedings of the
National Academy of Sciences 91: 4427–4430, 1994.
Burr, M. L. Effects of changes in fat, fish, and fibre intakes
on death and myocardial reinfarction: diet and reinfarction trial (Dart). Lancet, Sept. 757–761, 1989.
de Lorgeril, M. Mediterranean alpha-linolenic acid-rich
diet in secondary prevention of coronary heart disease.
Lancet 343: 1454–1459, 1994.
Harris, W. S. Modification of lipid-related atherosclerosis
risk factors by w–3 fatty acid ethyl esters in hyper-
triglyceridemic patients. J Nutr Biochem 4: 706–712,
1993.
Hibblein, J. R. Dietary polyunsaturated fatty acids and
depression: when cholesterol does not satisfy. American Journal of Clinical Nutrition 62(1): 1–9, 1995.

Kang, J. X. Antiarrhythmic effects of polyunsaturated fatty acids Recent Studies. Circulation 94: 1774–1780, 1996.

Kremer, J. M. Effects of modulation of inflammatory and immune parameters in patients with rheumatic and inflammatory disease receiving dietary supplemeation of n–3 and n–6 fatty acids. Lipids 31 Suppl: S243–7, 1996.

Leaf, A. Omega–3 fatty acids and prevention of ventricular fibrillation. Prosta Leuko Essen Fatty Acid 52: 197–198, 1995.

Stenson, W. F. Dietary supplementation with fish oil in ulcerative colitis. Annals of Internal Medicine 116: 609–614, 1992.

Stevens, L. J. Omega–3 fatty acids in boys with behavior, learning, and health problems. Physiol Behav 59 (4–5): 915–20, 1996.

GINGER

Bone, M. E. Ginger root—a new antiemetic. The effect of ginger root on postoperative nausea and vomiting after major gynecological surgery. Anaesthesia 45: 669–671, 1990.

Fischer-Rasmussen, W. Ginger treatment of hyperemesis gravidarum, European Journal of Obstetrics, Gynecology and Reproductive Biology 38: 19–24, 1990.

Fulder, S. Ginger as an anti-nausea remedy in pregnancy—the issue of safety. HerbalGram 38: 47, 1996. (American Botanical Council.)

Grontved, A. Ginger root against seasickness. A controlled trial on the open sea. Acta Otolaryngol (Stockh) 105: 45–49, 1988.

Mowrey, D. B. Motion Sickness, ginger and psychophysics. Lancet I: 655–657, 1982.

Pinco, R. G. European-American Phytomedicines Coalition Citizen Petition to Amend FDA's Monograph on Antiemetic Drug Products for Over-the-Counter ("OTC") Human Use to Include Ginger, May 26, 1995.

GINKGO

Itil, T. Natural substances in psychiatry (ginkgo biloba in dementia.). Psychopharmacology Bulletin 31: 147–158, 1995.

———. Early diagnosis and treatment of memory disturbances. American Journal of Electromedicine, June: 81–85, 1996.

Jung, F. Effect of gingko biloba on fluidity of blood and peripheral microcirculatiaon in volunteers. Arzneim-Forsch Drug Res 40: 589–593, 1990.

Hofferberth, B. The efficacy of EGb 761 in patients with senile dementia of the Alzheimer type, a double-blind, placebo-controlled study on different levels of investigation. Human Psychopharmacology 9: 215–22.

Hoyer, S. Possibilities and limits of therapy of cognition disorders in the elderly. Z Gerontol Geriatr 28(6): 457–62, 1995.

Huguet, F. Decreased cerebral 5-HTIA receptors during aging: reversal by ginkgo biloba extract (EGb 761). J. Pharm Pharmacol 46: 316–8, 1994.

Kanowski, S. Proof of efficacy of the ginkgo biloba special extract EGb 761 in outpatients suffering from mild to moderate primary degenerative dementia of the Alzheimer type or multi-infarct dementia. Pharmacopsychiatry 29 (2): 47–56, 1996.

Kleijnen, J. Ginkgo biloba for crebral insufficiency. British Journal of Clinical Pharmacology 34(4): 352–58, 1992.

Snowdon, D. A. Brain infarction and the clinical expression of Alzheimer disease. Journal of the American Medical Association 277: 813–817, 1997.

Sohn, M. Ginkgo biloba extract in the therapy of erectile dysfunction. J Sex Educ Ther 17: 53–61, 1991.

Vesper, J. Efficacy of ginkgo biloba in 90 outpatients with cerebral insufficiency caused by old age. Phytomedicine 1: 9–16, 1994.

GLUCOSAMINES

Crolle, G. Glucosamine sulphate for the management of arthrosis: a coantrolled clinical investigation. Current Medical Research and Opinion 7(2): 104–109, 1980.

Drovanti, A. Therapeutic activity of oral glucosamine sulfate in osteoarthrosis: a placebo-controlled double-blind investigation. Clinical Therapeutics 3: 260–72, 1980.

Muller-Fasbender, H. Glucosamine sulfate compared to ibuprofen in osteoarthritis of the knee. Osteoarthritis and Cartilage 2: 61–69, 1994.

Noack, W. Glucosamine sulfate in osteoarthritis of the knee, Osteoarthritis and Cartilage 2: 51–59, 1994.

Rovati, L.C. A large randomized, placebo controlled, double blind study of glucosamine sulfate vs. piroxicam and vs. their association, on the kinetics of the symptomatic effect in knee osteoarthritis. Osteoarthritis and Cartilage 2 (Suppl 1): 56, 1994.

Rovati, L. C. Clinical research in osteoarthritis: design and results of short-term and long-term trials with disease-modifying drugs. Int. J Tiss. Reac XIV (5): 243–251, 1992.

Vaz, A. L. Double-blind clinical evaluation of the relative efficacy of ibuprofen and glucosamine sulfate in the management of osteoarthrosis of the knee in out patients. Current Medical Research and Opinion 8: 145–9, 1982.

GRAPEFRUIT FIBER

Backey, P. A. Grapefruit pectin inhibits hypercholesterolemia and atherosclerosis in miniature swine. Clinical Cardiology 11: 595–600, 1988.

Baig, M. Pectin: Its interaction with serum lipoproteins. American Journal of Clinical Nutrition 34: 50–53, 1981.

Cerda, J. J. Inhibition of ahterosclerosis by dietary pectin in microswine with sustained hypercholesterolemia. Circulation 89: 1247–1253, 1994.

———. The effects of grapefruit pectin on patiets at risk for coronary heart disease without altering diet or lifestyle. Clinical Cardiology 11: 589–594, 1988.

KAVA

Bone, K. Kava—a safe herbal treatment for anxiety. British Journal of Phytotherapy 3 (4): 147–153. 1993/94.

Gebner B. Extract of kava-kava rhizome in comparison with diazepam and placebo. Zeitschrift für Phytother 15: 30–7, 1994

Herberg, K. W. Effect of kava-special extract WS 1490 combined with ethyl alcohol on safety relevant performance parameters. Blutalkohol 30: 96–105, 1993.

Kinzler, E. Effect of a special kava extract in patients with anxiety syndrome; a double blind placebo-controlled study over four weeks. Arzneimittel Forschung 41: 584–88, 1991.

Lehmann, E. Efficacy of a special kava extract (Piper methysticum) in patients with states of anxiety, tension and excitedness of non-mental origin—a double blind placebo-controlled study of four weeks treatment. Phytomedicine 3: 113–9, 1996.

Lindenberg, D. L-Kavain in comparison with oxazepam in anxiety disorders. A double blind study of clinical effectiveness. Fortschr Med 108: 49–50, 1990.

Munte, T. F. Effects of Oxazepam and an extract of kava roots on event-related potentials in a word recognition task. Neuropsychobiology 27: 46–53, 1993.

Warnecke, G. Psychosomatic Dysfunctions in the Female Climacteric. Fortschr Med 109: 119–22, 1991.

KUDZU

Keung, W. M. Therapeutic lessons from traditional Oriental medicine to contermpory Occidental pharmacology. in Toward a Molecular Basis of Alcohol Use and Abuse, edited by B. Jansson, et al. 1994 Birkhauser Verlag, Basel, Switzerland.

———. Daidzin and daidzein suppress free choice ethanol intake by Syrian golden hamsters, Proceedings of the National Academy of Sciences 90: 10008–10012, 1993.

Overstreet, D. H. Suppression of alcohol intake after adminstration of the Chinese herbal medicine NPI–028 and its derivatives. Alcoholism Clinical and Experimental Research 20(2): 221–227, 1996

LICORICE

Armanini, D. Further studies on the mechanism of the mineralocorticoid action of licorice in humans. Journal of Endocrinol Invest 19 (9): 624–9, 1996.

Baschetti, R. Chronic fatigue syndrome and neurally mediated hypotension. Journal of the American Medical Association 275: 359, 1996.

————. Chronic fatigue syndrome and liquorice. New Zealand Medical Journal, April 26, 157–158, 1995.

Borst, J. G. G. Synergistic action of liquorice and cortisone in Addison's and Simmonds' disease. Lancet 1: 657–663, 1953.

Bou-Holaigah, I. The relationship between neurally mediated hypotension and the chronic fatigue syndrome. Journal of the American Medical Association 274: 961–967, 1995.

Cleare, A. J. Contrasting neuroendocrine responses in depression and chronic fatigue syndrome. Journal of Affective Disorders 35: 283–289, 1995.

Demitrack, M. A. Evidence for impaired activation of the hypothalamic-pituitary-adrenal axis in patients with chronic fatigue syndrome. Journal of Clinical Endocrinology and Metabolism 73: 1224–34, 1991.

MILK THISTLE

Albrecht, M. Therapy of toxic liver pathologies with Legalon. Z Klin Med 47 (2): 87–92, 1992.

Buzzelli, G. A pilot study on the liver protective effect of silybin-phosphatidylcholine complex (IdB1016) in chronic active hepatitis. Int J Clin Pharmacol Ther Toxicol 31: 456–60, 1993.

Feher, J. Liver protecive action of silymarin therapy in chronic alcoholic liver diseases. Orv Hetil 130 (51): 2723–7, 1989.

Ferenci, R. Randomized controlled trial of silymarin treatment in patients with cirrhosis of the liver. J Hepatol 9: 105–113, 1989.

Fintelmann, A. The therapeutic activity of Legalon in toxic hepatic disorders demonstrated in a double blind trial. Therapiewoche 30: 5589–5594, 1980

Grossman, M. Spontaneous Regression of hepatocellular carcinoma. American Journal of Gastroenterology 90 (9): 1500–1503, 1995.

Kiesewetter, E. Results of two double-blind studies on the effect of silymarin in chronic hepatitis. Leber Magen Darm 7: 318–323, 1977.

Mascarella, S. Therapeutic and antilipoperoxidant effects of silybin-phosphatidylcholine complex in chronic liver disease: Preliminary result. Current Therapeutic Research 53 (1): 98–102, 1993.

Muzes, G. Effect of the bioflavonoid silymarin on the in vitro activity and expression of superoxide dismutase (SOD) enzyme. Acta Physiol Hung 78: 3–9, 1991.

Palasciano, G. The effect of silymarin on plasma levels of malon-dialdehyde in patients receiving long term treatment with psychotropic drugs. Current Therapeutic Research 55 (5): May, 1994: 537–545.

Szilard, S. Protective effect of Legalon in workers exposed to organic solvents. Acta Med Hung 45 (2): 249–56, 1988.

Vogel, G.. A Peculiarity among the flavonoids—silymarin, a compound active on the liver, a lecture. Proceedings of the International Bioflavonoid Symposium, Munich, 1981.

Yakhontova, O. I. Treatment of chronic liver diseases with hepatoprotectants . Vrachebnoe delo (Medicine) 5: 18–21, 1990.

OPC (GRAPE SEED AND PYCNOGENOL)

Blaszo, G. Oedemia-inhibiting effects of procyanidin. Acta Physiologica Academiae Hungaricae, Tomus 65 (2): 235–240, 1980.

Bombardelli, E. Vitis vinifera L. Fitoterapia, vol. lxvi (4): 291–317, 1995.

Corbe, C. Light vision and chorioretinal circulatiion. Study of the effect of procyanidolic oligomers (Endotelon). J Fr Ophtalmol 11(5): 453–60, 1988.

Delacroix, P. A double blind study of Endotelon in chronic venous insufficiency. La Revue de Medicine 27–28 August 31–September 7, 1981.

Thebaut, J. F. A study of Endotelon on the functional manifestations of venous insufficiency. A double blind study of 92 patients. Gazette Medicale 92, no. 12, 1985.

Lagrue, G. A study of the effects of procyanidol oligomers on capillary resistance in hypertension and in certain nephropathies. Sem Hop 57(33–36): 399–401, 1981.

Masquelier, J. Stabilisation du collagene par les oligomeres procyanidoliques, Acta Therapeutica 7: 101–105, 1981.

Robert, L. The effect of procyanidolic oligomers on vascular permeability. Pathol Biol (Paris); 38 (6): 608–16, 1990.

Rong, Y. Pycnogenol protects vascular endothelial cells from t-butyl hydroperoxide induced oxidant injury. Biotechnol Ther 5(3–4): 117–26, 1994.

PEPPERMINT OIL

Dew, M. J. Peppermint oil for the irritable bowel syndrome: a multicentre trial. British Journal of Clinical Practice 38: 394–98, 1984.

Gobel, H. Effectiveness of Oleum menthae piperitae and paracetamol in therapy of headachc of the tension type. Nervenarzt 67 (8): 672–81, 1996.

———. Effect of peppermint and eucalyptus oil preparations on neurophysiological and experimental algesimetric headache parameters. Cephalalgia 14(3): 228–34, 1994.

Leicester, R. Peppermint oil to reduce colonic spasm during endoscopy. Lancet II: 989, 1982.

Somerville, K. Delayed release peppermint capsules (Colpermin) for the spastic colon syndrome: a pharmacolkinetic study. Br. J Clin Pharmacol 18: 638–640, 1984.

Rees, W. Treating irritable bowel syndrome with peppermint oil. Br. Med J. II: 835–36, 1979.

SAW PALMETTO

Boccafoschi, C. Confronto fra estratto di serenoa repens e placebo mediate prova clinica controllata in pazienti con adenomatosi prostatica. Urologia 50: 1257–1268, 1983.

Braeckman, J. The extract of Serenoa repens in the treatment of benign prostatic hyperplasia: a multicenter open study. Current Therapeutic Research 55: 776–785, 1994.

Champault, A. Double blind trial of an extract of the plant Serenoa repens in benign prostate hyperplasia. British J. Clin Pharmacol 18: 461–462, 1984.

Emili, E. Risultani clinici su un nuovo farmaco nella terapia dell'ipertrofia della prostata (Permixon). Urologia 50: 1042–1048, 1983.

Murray, M. Saw palmetto extract vs. Proscar, the American Journal of Natural Medicine, 1(1): 8–9, 1994.

Vahlensieck, W., Jr. Benigne prostatahyperplasie— behandlung mit sabalfruchtestrakt. Fortschr Med 111: 323–326, 1993.

ST. JOHN'S WORT

Bladt, S. Inhibition of MAO by fractions and constituents of hypericum extract. Journal of Geriatric Psychiatry and Neurology 7(suppl 1): S57–59, 1994.

Bombardelli, E. Hypericum perforatum. Fitoterapia LXVI, (1): 43–68 1995

Harrer, G. Effectiveness and tolerance of the hypericum extract LI 160 compared to maprotiline: a multicenter double-blind study. Journal of Geriatric Psychiatry and Neurology 7(suppl 1): S24–28,1994.

Martinez, B. Hypericum in the treatment of seasonal affective disorders. Journal of Geriatric Psychiatry and Neurology 7(suppl 1): S29-S33,1994.

Perovic, S. Pharmacological profile of hypericum extract. Effect on serotonin uptake by postsynaptic receptors. Arzneimittelforschung 45(11): 1145–8, 1995.

Sommer, H. Placebo-controlled double-blind study examining the effectiveness of an hypericum preparation in 105 mildly depressed patients. Journal of Geriatric Psychiatry and Neurology 7(suppl 1): S9–11, 1994.

Vorbach, E.-U. Effectiveness and tolerance of the hypericum extract LI 160 in comparison with imipramine: randomized double-blind study with 135 outpatients. Journal of Geriatric Psychiatry and Neurology 7(suppl 1): S19–23, 1994.

Woelk, H. Benefits and risks of the hypericum extract LI 160: drug monitoring study with 3250 patients. Journal of Geriatric Psychiatry and Neurology 7(suppl 1): S34–38, 1994.

VALERIAN

Albrecht, M. Psychopharmaceuticals and safety in traffic. Zeits Allegmeinmed 71: 1215–1221, 1995.

Dressing, H. Insomnia: Are valerian/balm combinations of equal value to benzodiazepine? Therapiewoche 42: 726–736, 1992.

Leathwood, P. D. Aqueous extract of valerian reduces

latency to fall asleep in man. Planta Medica 54: 144–48, 1985.

————. Aqueous extract of valerian root improves sleep quality in man. Pharmacol Biochem Behav 17: 65–71, 1982.

Lindahl, O. Double blind study of a valerian preparation. Pharmacol Biochem Behav 32 (4): 1065–6, 1989.

Willey, Leanna B. Valerian Overdose: A Case Report. Veterinary and Human Toxicology 37 (4), August: 364–365, 1995.

VITAMINS C AND E

Azen, S. P. Effect of supplementary antioxidant vitamin intake on carotid arterial wall intima-media thickness in a controlled clinical trial of cholesterol lowering. Circulation 94 10: 2369–72, 1996.

Gatto, L. M. Ascorbic acid induces a favorable lipoprotein profile in women. Journal of the American College of Nutrition 15: 154–158, 1996.

Gokce, N. Basic research in antioxidant inhibition of steps in atherogenesis. Journal of Cardiovascular Risk 3(4): 352–7, 1996.

Hatch, G. E. Asthma, inhaled oxidants, and dietary antioxidants. American Journal of Clinical Nutrition 61 (suppl): 625S–30S, 1995.

Heitzer, T. Antioxidant vitamin C improves endothelial dysfunction in chronic smokers. Circulation 94: 6–9, 1996.

Levine, Glenn N. Ascorbic Acid Reverses Endothelial vasomotor dysfunction in patients with coronary artery disease. Circulation 93: 1107–1113, 1996.

Stephens, N. G. Randomised controlled trial of vitamin E in patients with coronary disease: Cambridge Heart

Antioxidant Study (CHAOS. Lancet 347(9004): 781–6, 1996.

Tomoda, H. Possible prevention of postangioplasty restenosis by ascorbic acid. American Journal of Cardiology 78 (11): 1284–1286, 1996.

Verlangieri, A. Effects of a-tocopherol supplementation on experimentally induced primate atherosclerosis. Journal of American College of Nutrition. 11(2): 130–37, 1992.

Weber, C. Increased adhesiveness of isolated monocytes to endothelium is prevented by vitamin C intake in smokers. Circulation 93: 1488–1492, 1996.

TO CONTACT THE AUTHOR

If you use the natural remedies described in this book or use other natural remedies not included in this book, and want to tell the author about your experience, you can write to: Miracle Cures, P.O. Box 311, Waynesboro, PA 17268.

INDEX